INTERMITTENT FASTING GUIDE AND COOKBOOK FOR WOMEN OVER 50

1000 Days Of Delicious Intermittent Fasting Recipes And The Complete Guide To Help With Menopause, Regain Vitality And Love Yourself.

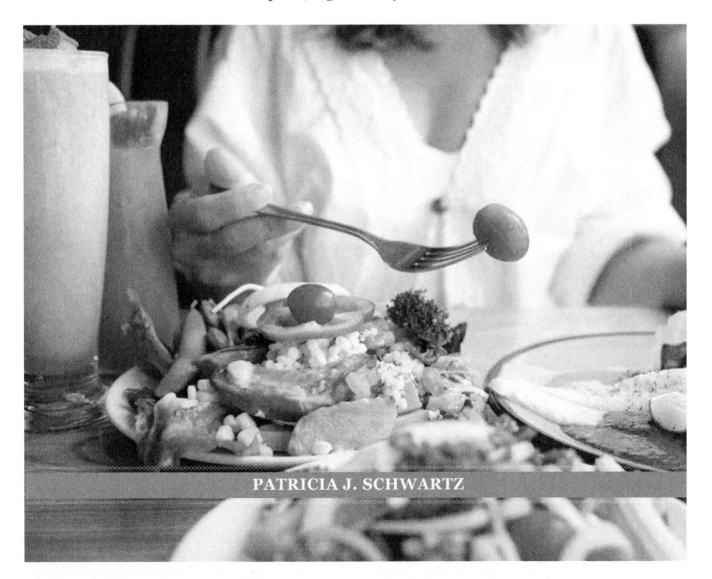

PATRICIA J. SCHWARTZ

EDITOR: LYN

INTERIOR DESIGN: FAIZAN

COVER ART: ABR

FOOD STYLIST: JO

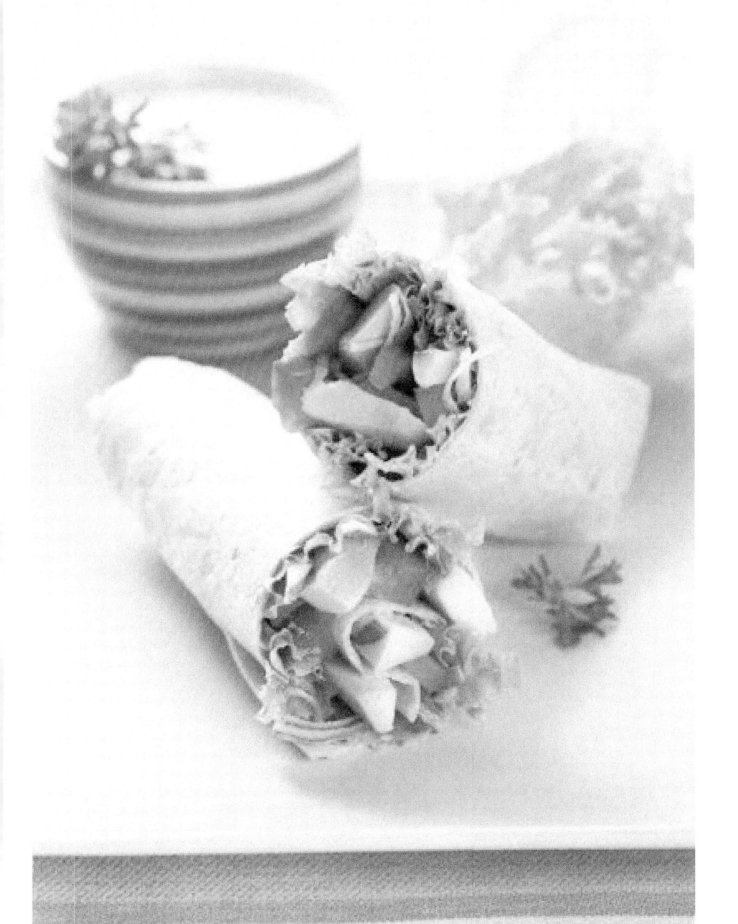

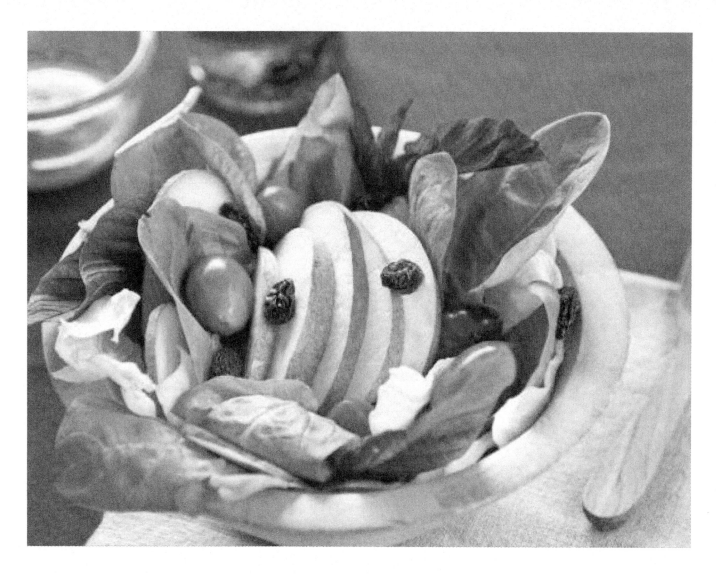

Table of Contents

Introduction

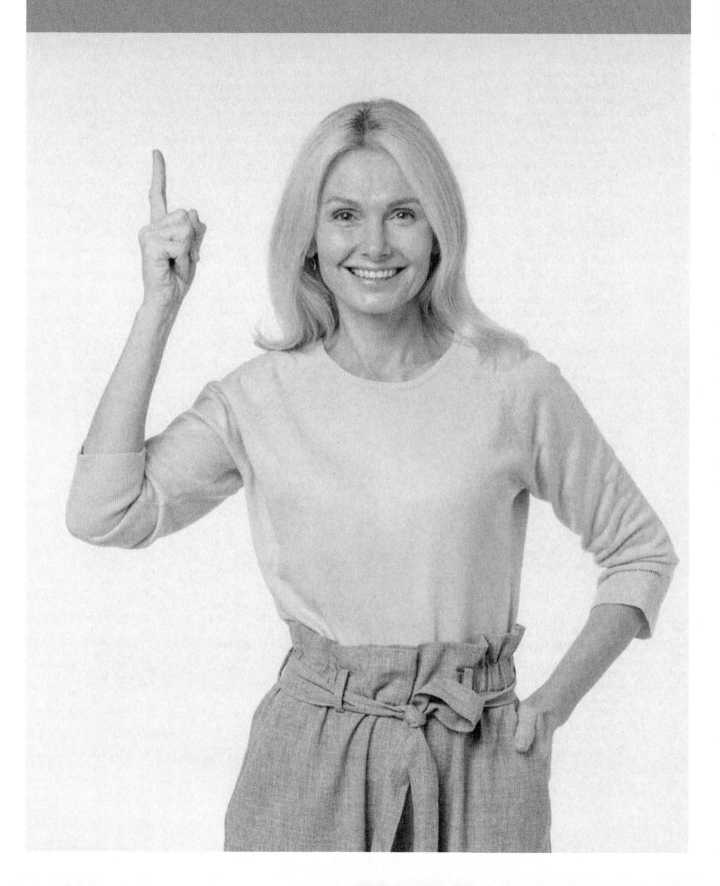

Oh seeker of truth, listen to me,
About a practice that can set you free,
Intermittent fasting, a method of old,
To purify body, mind, and soul.

It is not about depriving yourself of food,
But about finding balance, in the right mood,
For when you fast, your body heals,
And your spirit soars, as your ego kneels.

No need to starve, just control your pace,
Skip a meal or two, and give your gut a break,
And see how your body reacts with grace,
As toxins leave and health starts to wake.

And as you fast, let your mind be still,
Reflect on life, and seek divine will,
For this is not just a physical act,
But a journey within, that can impact.

So embrace intermittent fasting with an open heart,
And let it guide you to a healthier start,
For when your body and spirit align,
You'll find peace, joy, and purpose divine.

Chapter 1
Basics of Intermittent Fasting

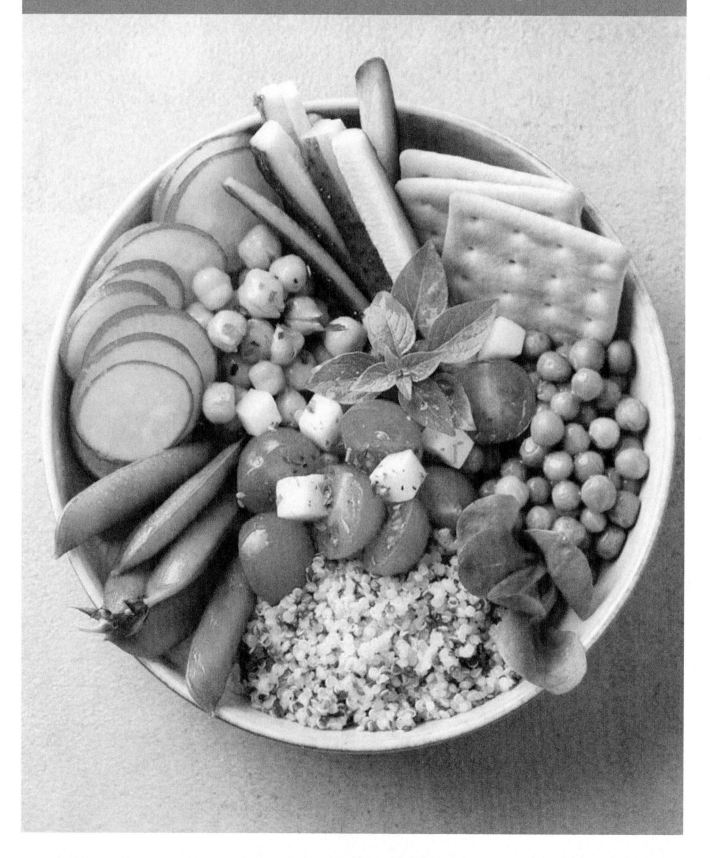

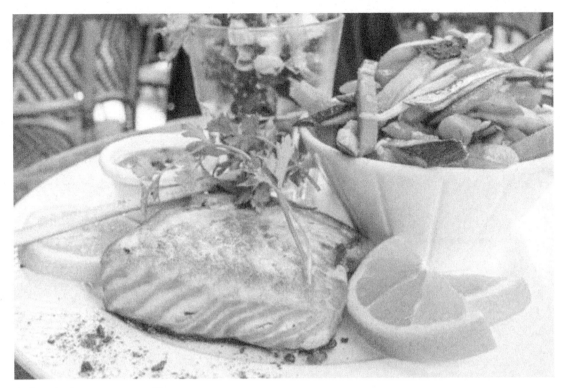

What Is Intermittent Fasting

Intermittent fasting is a dietary practice that involves cycling between periods of eating and periods of abstaining from food. It is not about what you eat but rather when you eat. There are different ways to practice intermittent fasting, such as the 16/8 method, where you eat during an 8-hour window and fast for the remaining 16 hours, or the 5:2 method, where you eat normally for five days and limit your calorie intake to 500-600 calories for two non-consecutive days.

Intermittent fasting has been shown to have several health benefits, including weight loss, improved insulin sensitivity, reduced inflammation, and improved brain function. It can also promote longevity by activating cellular repair processes and reducing oxidative stress. When you fast, your body's insulin levels decrease, which allows stored fat to be released and used for energy. This can lead to weight loss and improved metabolic health. Additionally, fasting triggers a process called autophagy, where your body breaks down and recycles old cells and proteins, which can have anti-aging and disease-fighting benefits.

However, it is important to note that intermittent fasting may not be suitable for everyone, especially those with certain medical conditions or women who are pregnant or breastfeeding. It is always recommended to consult a healthcare professional before starting any new diet or fasting regimen.

History of Intermittent Fasting

YOU MIGHT THINK THAT IF IS A NEW METHOD, BUT THAT'S NOT TRUE.

Intermittent fasting is not a new concept and has been practiced for thousands of years in different cultures and religions. The ancient Greeks, for example, practiced a form of intermittent fasting, where they would fast for 24 hours before competing in the Olympic Games. Many religious traditions also incorporate fasting as a spiritual practice, such as Ramadan for Muslims, Yom Kippur for Jews, and Lent for Christians.

In modern times, intermittent fasting gained popularity as a weight loss and health-promoting strategy in the early 1900s. In the 1930s, researchers discovered that calorie restriction could increase the lifespan of laboratory animals, which led to further studies on the benefits of fasting. However, it wasn't until the 21st century that intermittent fasting became a mainstream health trend, with the publication of books like "The Fast Diet" by Dr. Michael Mosley and "The 8-Hour Diet" by David Zinczenko.

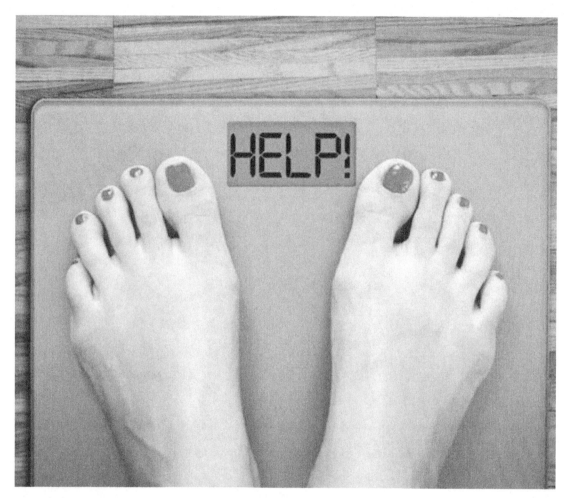

Today, intermittent fasting has become a popular approach to weight loss and overall health, with different variations of fasting schedules and methods being promoted by health experts and celebrities alike.

The Science of Intermittent Fasting

The science behind intermittent fasting is still evolving, but recent research has shed light on some of the physiological mechanisms that may contribute to its health benefits.

One of the primary ways that intermittent fasting can promote weight loss is by reducing overall calorie intake. By limiting the window of time during which you can eat, you may naturally consume fewer calories over the course of the day, which can lead to a calorie deficit and subsequent weight loss.

Intermittent fasting also appears to have metabolic benefits. During fasting periods, the body shifts from burning glucose for energy to burning fat, which can lead to improved insulin sensitivity and a reduction in inflammation. This metabolic shift may also trigger a process called autophagy, where the body breaks down and recycles old or damaged cells, leading to cellular repair and renewal.

Additionally, some studies have suggested that intermittent fasting may have anti-aging effects by protecting against age-related diseases such as diabetes, heart disease, and cancer. This may be due to the reduction in oxidative stress and inflammation that occurs during fasting periods.

WEIGHT LOSS

weight loss is one of the primary goals of intermittent fasting for many people. By reducing overall calorie intake and promoting fat burning, intermittent fasting can create a calorie deficit that leads to weight loss over time. However, it's important to remember that weight loss is not the only benefit of intermittent fasting and that the scientific evidence on its long-term weight loss effects is still evolving. Other potential benefits of intermittent fasting include improved metabolic health, reduced inflammation, and cellular repair and renewal. It's always recommended to consult a healthcare professional before starting an intermittent fasting regimen and to approach weight loss as part of a broader approach to overall health and wellness.

MUSCLE BUILDING

There is some evidence to suggest that fasting can increase the production of human growth hormone (HGH) in the body, although the extent of this increase and its health effects are still debated among researchers.

Some studies have shown that fasting for short periods of time can lead to an increase in HGH production, which may have benefits for muscle growth, fat burning, and anti-aging. For example, one study found that a 24-hour fast led to a 2000% increase in HGH levels in men and a 1300% increase in women. Another study found that HGH levels increased by 1250% after just a week of fasting.

REDUCED DIABETES RISK

intermittent fasting may help improve insulin sensitivity by regulating insulin levels in the body. When you eat, your body releases insulin to help process the glucose from the food and store it as energy. However, if you constantly eat throughout the day, your body may become less sensitive to insulin over time, which can lead to insulin resistance and the development of type 2 diabetes.

Intermittent fasting can help prevent this by limiting the window of time during which you eat, which can help regulate insulin levels and prevent insulin resistance. By creating periodic lows and highs of insulin in the body, intermittent fasting may also help improve glucose control and prevent spikes in blood sugar levels.

ELEVATED BRAIN PERFORMANCE

One potential way that intermittent fasting may improve brain function is by promoting the production of a protein called brain-derived neurotrophic factor (BDNF), which is involved in the growth and maintenance of neurons in the brain. Studies have shown that fasting can increase BDNF levels, which may have benefits for learning, memory, and mood.

Intermittent fasting may also have neuroprotective effects by reducing oxidative stress and inflammation in the brain, which can contribute to age-related cognitive decline and neurodegenerative diseases such as Alzheimer's and Parkinson's. Additionally, intermittent fasting has been shown to promote the production of ketones, which are a source of energy for the brain and may have neuroprotective effects.

Foods To Eat

LEAN PROTEINS

proteins can take longer to digest than carbohydrates or fats, the idea that proteins take one to two days to digest completely is a bit of an exaggeration. In reality, the digestion and absorption of proteins can vary depending on a number of factors, including the type and source of the protein, how it's prepared, and individual differences in metabolism.

That said, including lean proteins in your eating window during intermittent fasting can be beneficial for a number of reasons. Proteins are important for building and repairing tissues in the body, including muscle tissue, and can help you feel full and satisfied between meals. Lean proteins, such as chicken, fish, and legumes, are also typically lower in calories and fat than other sources of protein, making them a good choice for weight management.

FRUITS

Consuming fruits during the eating window of intermittent fasting can provide a source of vitamins and minerals that can help support overall health and metabolism during the fasting period.

Fruits are a good source of important vitamins and minerals, such as vitamin C, potassium, and fiber, which play important roles in maintaining a healthy metabolism. Vitamin C, for example, is an antioxidant that helps protect cells from damage and is involved in collagen synthesis, which is important for healthy skin and connective tissues. Potassium is an essential mineral that helps regulate fluid balance, nerve function, and muscle contractions. Fiber is important for digestive health and can help promote feelings of fullness and satiety.

It's worth noting, however, that fruits also contain natural sugars, which can raise blood sugar levels and potentially break the fast if consumed in large amounts. It's recommended to choose fruits that are lower in sugar, such as berries, and to consume them in moderation during the eating window.

VEGETABLES

Incorporating vegetables into the eating window of intermittent fasting can provide a variety of health benefits. Vegetables are rich in important nutrients, including vitamins, minerals, and fiber, which can help support overall health and well-being.

Eating a diet rich in vegetables has been associated with a reduced risk of chronic diseases such as heart disease, type 2 diabetes, and certain types of cancer. This is thought to be due in part to the antioxidant and anti-inflammatory properties of many vegetables, which can help protect cells from damage and reduce inflammation in the body.

Vegetables are also important for brain health, as they contain a variety of nutrients that support cognitive function and may help protect against age-related cognitive decline. For example, leafy greens such as spinach and kale are rich in folate, a B vitamin that is important for brain health, while cruciferous vegetables like broccoli and cauliflower contain compounds that may have neuroprotective effects.

When incorporating vegetables into the eating window of intermittent fasting, it's important to choose a variety of colors and types to ensure that you're getting a range of nutrients. It's also recommended to consume vegetables that are low in calories and carbohydrates, such as leafy greens, broccoli, and peppers, to help support weight management and avoid breaking the fast.

WATER

Water is indeed a crucial component of intermittent fasting, as it helps support hydration and can help promote feelings of fullness and satiety during the fasting period.

When following an intermittent fasting regimen, it's important to stay well-hydrated throughout the day, as dehydration can lead to a variety of symptoms, including headaches, fatigue, and difficulty concentrating. Drinking plenty of water can also help promote feelings of fullness and satiety, which can make it easier to stick to the fasting schedule.

In addition to water, other non-caloric beverages such as herbal tea and black coffee can also be consumed during the fasting period. These beverages can help provide a source of hydration and can also help curb hunger and promote mental alertness.

It's important to note, however, that sugary or artificially sweetened beverages should be avoided during the fasting period, as they can raise blood sugar levels and potentially break the fast. It's also important to consume water and other beverages in moderation, as consuming large amounts at once can potentially disrupt electrolyte balance and lead to other health issues.

BONE BROTH

Bone broth is a nutrient-dense food that can be a valuable addition to the eating window of intermittent fasting. It is made by simmering animal bones and connective tissue, such as chicken or beef bones, for an extended period of time to extract the minerals, collagen, and other nutrients.

Bone broth is rich in vitamins and minerals, including calcium, magnesium, and phosphorus, which are important for bone health and overall health and well-being. It also contains collagen and gelatin, which can help support healthy skin, hair, and nails.

In addition, bone broth is a good source of protein, which can help support muscle maintenance and repair during the fasting period. Consuming a small amount of protein during the eating window of intermittent fasting can help promote feelings of fullness and satiety, which can make it easier to stick to the fasting schedule.

It's important to note, however, that bone broth does contain calories, so it should be consumed in moderation during the eating window to avoid breaking the fast. It's also important to choose bone broth that is made with high-quality ingredients and to avoid products that contain added sugars or artificial ingredients.

Foods To Avoid

Chips, Cookies, Candies, and Cakes

Bakery items such as cakes, cookies, and pastries are typically high in refined carbohydrates and added sugars, which can cause a rapid spike in blood glucose and insulin levels. For this reason, it is generally recommended to avoid these foods during the fasting period of intermittent fasting.

Consuming high amounts of processed sugars and refined carbohydrates can lead to fluctuations in blood sugar levels, which can cause feelings of fatigue, irritability, and hunger. Additionally, consuming these types of foods can lead to insulin resistance over time, which can increase the risk of developing chronic health conditions such as type 2 diabetes and heart disease.

Instead, it's recommended to consume nutrient-dense foods during the eating window of intermittent fasting, such as lean proteins, fruits, vegetables, whole grains, and healthy fats. These foods provide sustained energy and can help promote feelings of fullness and satiety, making it easier to stick to the fasting schedule.

FRUIT DRINKS

Fruit drinks, especially those that are commercially produced, are often high in added sugars and food concentrates, which can make them very high in sugar and calories. For this reason, it is generally advised to avoid fruit drinks during the fasting period of intermittent fasting.

Consuming high amounts of sugar, whether from fruit drinks or other sources, can cause a rapid spike in blood glucose levels, leading to an increase in insulin levels and potential insulin resistance over time. Additionally, consuming high amounts of sugar can contribute to weight gain and an increased risk of chronic health conditions, such as type 2 diabetes and heart disease.
Instead of fruit drinks, it's recommended to consume whole fruits during the eating window of intermittent fasting. Whole fruits are a good source of vitamins, minerals, and fiber, and they contain natural sugars that are less likely to cause rapid fluctuations in blood sugar levels.

HIGHLY SWEETENED TEAS AND COFFEES

Sweetened coffee and tea beverages are often high in added sugars, which can make them very high in calories and disrupt the fasting period of intermittent fasting. For this reason, it is generally advised to avoid sweetened coffee and tea during the fasting period.

Consuming high amounts of added sugars can cause a rapid rise in blood glucose levels, leading to an increase in insulin levels and potential insulin resistance over time. Additionally, consuming high amounts of added sugars can contribute to weight gain and an increased risk of chronic health conditions, such as type 2 diabetes and heart disease.

Instead of sweetened coffee and tea, it's recommended to consume plain coffee or tea during the fasting period of intermittent fasting. Black coffee and tea are low in calories and can provide a natural energy boost without disrupting the fasting period.

SUGARY CEREALS

Sugary cereals are typically composed of refined grains and high amounts of added sugars, which can make them a poor choice for overall health and for the fasting period of intermittent fasting.

Refined grains have been processed to remove the bran and germ, which also removes important nutrients such as fiber, vitamins, and minerals. Consuming high amounts of refined grains and added sugars can cause a rapid rise in blood glucose levels, leading to an increase in insulin levels and potential insulin resistance over time. Additionally, consuming high amounts of added sugars can contribute to weight gain and an increased risk of chronic health conditions, such as type 2 diabetes and heart disease.

Instead of sugary cereals, it's recommended to consume whole-grain cereals that are low in added sugars and high in fiber during the eating window of intermittent fasting. Whole-grain cereals provide important nutrients and can help to keep you feeling full and satisfied for longer periods of time.

Chapter 2
Intermittent Fasting For Women

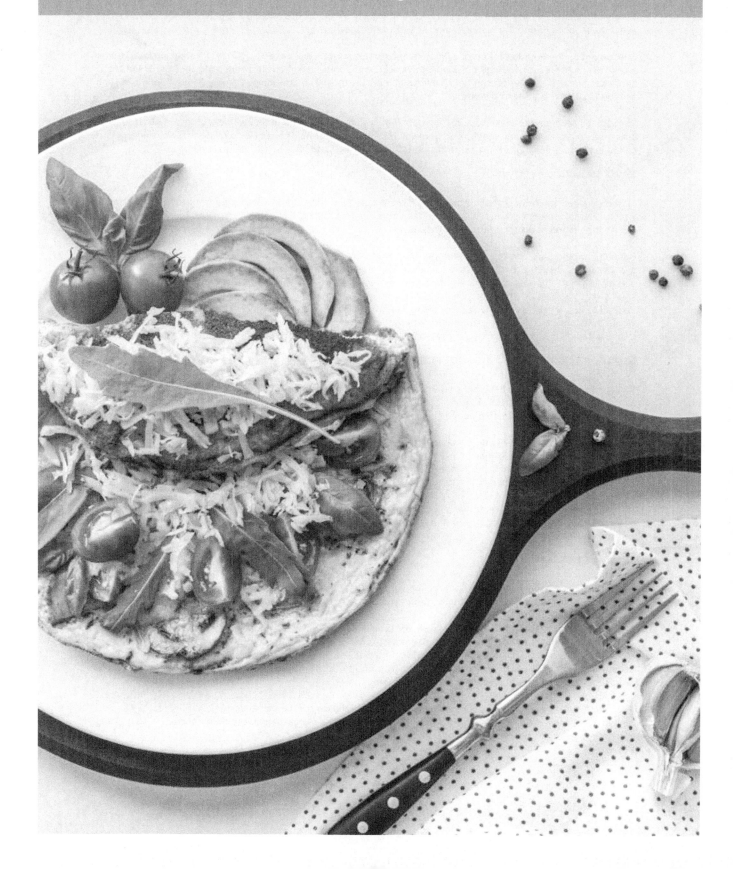

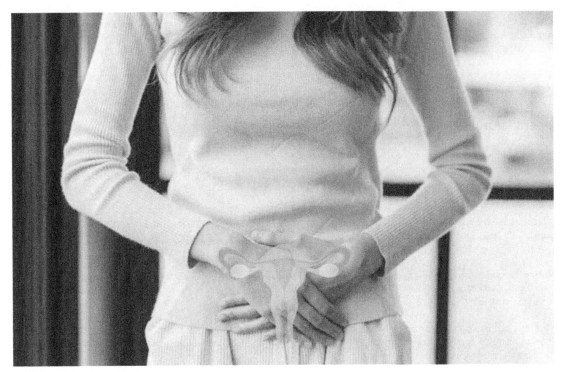

Changes Faced By Women over 50

PERIMENOPAUSE

Perimenopause is a natural phase of life that many women experience as they approach their midlife years. It can be a challenging time, as the body undergoes a range of hormonal changes that can cause a variety of symptoms.

For me, perimenopause has been a rollercoaster ride of hot flashes, mood swings, and unpredictable periods. It's like my body is playing a game of roulette, with no clear pattern or predictability to what's going to happen next.

One day I'll be feeling fine, and the next day I'm sweating through my clothes and feeling like I'm on an emotional rollercoaster. It can be frustrating, exhausting, and downright confusing at times.

But despite the challenges, I've learned to embrace this phase of life as a time of transition and growth. It's a time to reflect on my past and prepare for the future, to take stock of my health and well-being, and to focus on self-care and self-love.

Through it all, I remind myself that I'm not alone. Millions of women around the world are experiencing perimenopause, and there's a growing body of research and resources available to help us navigate this journey.

MENOPAUSE

Menopause is a natural transition that many women experience as they approach their midlife years. It's a time when the body undergoes significant hormonal changes, and it can bring about a range of physical and emotional symptoms.

For me, menopause has been a time of mixed emotions. On one hand, I feel relieved that I no longer have to deal with the uncertainty and unpredictability of perimenopause. On the other hand, I'm also aware that my body is going through a significant change, and that can be scary and overwhelming at times.

The physical symptoms of menopause can vary from woman to woman, but for me, hot flashes and night sweats have been the most challenging. I can be going about my day, feeling perfectly fine, and then suddenly I'm drenched in sweat and feeling like I'm on fire. It can be embarrassing and disruptive, and it's definitely not a topic that's easy to discuss with others.

But despite the challenges, I'm also aware that menopause is a time of empowerment and transformation. It's a time to embrace my inner wisdom and strength, to focus on my health and well-being, and to prioritize my own needs and desires.

I'm grateful for the support and resources that are available to me, whether it's through my healthcare provider, online communities, or friends and family who have gone through this transition themselves. I know that I'm not alone, and that there are many other women out there who are going through the same thing.

POSTMENOPAUSE

Postmenopause is a phase of life that comes after menopause, and it can last for many years. During this time, our hormone levels have typically stabilized, and we may experience a range of changes and challenges related to aging.

One of the most notable changes that many women experience in postmenopause is a gradual loss of bone density. This can increase the risk of osteoporosis and fractures, which can impact our mobility and quality of life. To support bone health, it's important to focus on a diet that's rich in calcium, vitamin D, and other key nutrients, as well as engaging in weight-bearing exercise.

Other common symptoms of postmenopause can include vaginal dryness and atrophy, which can lead to discomfort and pain during sex. This can be managed with various treatments, including topical creams, hormone therapy, and lubricants.

Postmenopause can also be a time when women experience changes in their mental health, such as an increased risk of depression or anxiety. It's important to prioritize self-care and seek support from loved ones or healthcare providers if needed.

Overall, postmenopause is a time when many women may feel more comfortable and confident in their bodies and lives, but it can also come with unique challenges. By prioritizing our health and well-being, staying connected to our bodies and loved ones, and seeking support when needed, we can navigate this phase of life with grace and resilience.

Why Women over 50 Should Do Intermittent Fasting?

Intermittent fasting can be beneficial for women over 50 for a number of reasons. Here are a few:

Weight management: As we age, it can become more difficult to maintain a healthy weight. Intermittent fasting can help with weight management by limiting the amount of time we have to eat, which can lead to consuming fewer calories overall.

Hormonal balance: Hormonal changes are common in women over 50, and these changes can impact our metabolism and weight. Intermittent fasting has been shown to improve insulin sensitivity, which can help balance hormones and support overall health.

Brain health: As we age, cognitive decline can become a concern. Intermittent fasting has been shown to have neuroprotective effects, potentially reducing the risk of cognitive decline and Alzheimer's disease.

Cardiovascular health: Heart disease is a common concern for women over 50. Intermittent fasting has been shown to have a positive impact on various cardiovascular risk factors, such as blood pressure, cholesterol levels, and inflammation.

Longevity: Intermittent fasting has been linked to increased longevity and a reduced risk of age-related diseases.

Is It Safe?

Intermittent fasting can be safe for women over 50 when done correctly and under the guidance of a healthcare provider. However, it's important to note that there is no "one-size-fits-all" approach to intermittent fasting, and what works for one person may not work for another.

Women over 50 may have unique health concerns and considerations, such as hormonal changes, chronic health conditions, and medication use. These factors should be taken into account when determining whether intermittent fasting is appropriate.

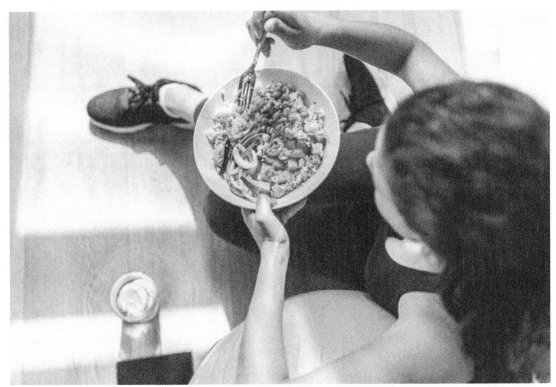

It's also important to approach intermittent fasting with a balanced and nutritious diet. Women over 50 may require different levels of certain nutrients, such as protein and calcium, to support bone health and muscle mass.

People who should consult with a healthcare professional before fasting intermittently

DIABETES TYPE 1 PATIENT

It is strongly recommended that people with Type 1 diabetes consult with a healthcare professional before attempting intermittent fasting. Type 1 diabetes is a chronic condition in which the body does not produce insulin, a hormone needed to regulate blood sugar levels. Intermittent fasting can cause fluctuations in blood sugar levels, which can be dangerous for people with Type 1 diabetes.

People with Type 1 diabetes must carefully monitor their blood sugar levels and adjust their insulin doses accordingly. Intermittent fasting can make it difficult to manage blood sugar levels, especially if the eating window is too short or if the person consumes too much food during the feeding window.

A healthcare professional can provide guidance on how to safely and effectively approach intermittent fasting while managing Type 1 diabetes. They may recommend adjusting insulin doses, monitoring blood sugar levels more frequently, or modifying the length of the fasting and feeding windows.

People suffering from eating disorders and psychological issues

It is strongly recommended that individuals with a history of eating disorders or psychological issues consult with a healthcare professional before attempting intermittent fasting. Intermittent fasting can be challenging for some people, particularly those with a history of disordered eating or psychological conditions such as anxiety or depression.

Intermittent fasting may trigger feelings of deprivation or restriction in individuals with a history of eating disorders, which could lead to disordered eating behaviors. It can also trigger anxiety or depression in some individuals, particularly if they have a history of mental health issues.

A healthcare professional can provide guidance on how to safely and effectively approach intermittent fasting while managing any underlying psychological issues or eating disorders. They may recommend an individualized approach that takes into account the individual's medical and psychological history, as well as their nutritional needs.

People who start developing serious side effects every time they try IF

It is recommended that individuals who experience serious side effects when attempting intermittent fasting consult with a healthcare professional. While intermittent fasting can have many potential benefits, it may not be suitable for everyone. Some people may experience side effects such as fatigue, headaches, dizziness, or nausea when fasting, particularly if they are new to the practice or have underlying medical conditions.

A healthcare professional can help determine whether intermittent fasting is a safe and appropriate approach for an individual based on their medical history, current health status, and any medications they may be taking. They can also provide guidance on how to minimize potential side effects and support overall health and well-being during the fasting period.

It is important to note that anyone who experiences severe or persistent side effects while fasting should stop the practice immediately and seek medical attention. Symptoms such as severe abdominal pain, vomiting, or fainting should not be ignored and may require urgent medical attention.

IF Mistakes And How To Avoid Them

STARTING DRASTICALLY WITH IF

Starting drastically with intermittent fasting can be a mistake because it can lead to several negative side effects, such as headaches, dizziness, fatigue, and irritability. When you abruptly change your eating habits and go without food for extended periods, your body may struggle to adjust to the new routine, leading to unpleasant symptoms.

To avoid this mistake, it is recommended to start with a gradual approach to intermittent fasting. For example, instead of jumping straight into a 16-hour fasting window, you could start with a shorter fasting window, such as 12 hours, and gradually increase the duration over time. This allows your body to adjust to the new routine and can help minimize any negative side effects.

It is also important to ensure that you are getting adequate nutrition during the eating window. Eating a balanced diet with plenty of fruits, vegetables, lean proteins, and healthy fats can help ensure that your body is getting the nutrients it needs to support optimal health and well-being.

Additionally, staying well hydrated and getting enough sleep can also help support your body during the fasting period. Drinking plenty of water and avoiding excessive caffeine or alcohol consumption can help minimize dehydration and other negative side effects.

Overall, it is important to approach intermittent fasting with a gradual and balanced approach to minimize the risk of negative side effects and maximize the potential benefits of this practice.

CHOOSING THE WRONG FASTING PLAN

Choosing the wrong fasting plan is a mistake because it can result in negative side effects or failure to achieve the desired results. For example, someone who chooses a plan that involves very long fasting periods may experience intense hunger pangs or fatigue, making it difficult to sustain the plan long-term.

To avoid this mistake, it's important to research and understand different types of fasting plans before choosing one that suits your lifestyle, health status, and personal goals. It's recommended to start with a less restrictive plan, such as a 12:12 or 16:8 fasting schedule, before trying more advanced plans like alternate-day fasting or prolonged fasting.

Additionally, it's important to listen to your body and make adjustments as needed. If you are experiencing negative side effects like dizziness, fatigue, or intense hunger, it may be a sign that the fasting plan is not right for you.

To avoid these issues, you need to select a plan that fits your daily routine without affecting your working hours and sleep-wake cycle.

OVEREATING RIGHT AFTER YOU BREAK A FAST

Overeating right after breaking a fast is a mistake because it can negate the benefits of the fasting period and even cause digestive discomfort. When you fast, your body enters a state of calorie deficit, which can cause your stomach to shrink and your digestive system to slow down. If you eat a large meal right after breaking your fast, your body may not be prepared to handle the sudden influx of food, leading to bloating, indigestion, or even nausea.

To avoid this mistake, it's important to break your fast with a small, nutrient-dense meal and wait for a while before eating a larger meal. Start with something like a small serving of vegetables, a piece of fruit, or a light soup to ease your digestive system back into eating mode. Avoid foods that are high in sugar or refined carbohydrates, which can cause a sudden spike in blood sugar levels.

Also, it's important to eat slowly and mindfully, savoring each bite and paying attention to your body's hunger and fullness signals. If you feel satisfied after a small meal, wait for a while before eating more. Remember that the goal of intermittent fasting is not to deprive yourself of food, but to develop a healthier relationship with food and improve your overall health.

EATING TOO LITTLE BEFORE THE FASTING WINDOW

Eating too little before the fasting window is a mistake because it can cause several negative effects on the body. If you don't eat enough before starting your fast, your body may not have enough energy to sustain itself during the fasting period. This can lead to feelings of weakness, dizziness, and fatigue, which can make it difficult to carry out daily activities.

Additionally, not eating enough before the fasting window can lead to overeating during the eating period, which can undo the benefits of fasting. Overeating can cause blood sugar levels to spike, leading to insulin resistance and weight gain.

To avoid this mistake, it's important to consume a balanced and nutritious meal before the fasting window. The meal should include lean proteins, complex carbohydrates, and healthy fats to provide enough energy for the body to sustain itself during the fast.
It's also important to stay hydrated by drinking plenty of water throughout the day. This can help reduce feelings of hunger and keep the body functioning properly. Finally, it's important to listen to your body and adjust your eating habits accordingly. If you find yourself feeling weak or fatigued during the fast, it may be time to reassess your eating habits and adjust accordingly.

NOT DRINKING ENOUGH WATER

Not drinking enough water while doing intermittent fasting is a mistake because water is essential for numerous bodily functions, including digestion, elimination of toxins, and maintaining proper hydration levels. When fasting, it is essential to stay hydrated to avoid dehydration, which can lead to headaches, fatigue, and other unpleasant symptoms.

To avoid this mistake, it is important to make sure you are drinking enough water throughout the day, especially during your fasting window. It is recommended to drink at least 8 glasses of water per day, or more if you are physically active. You can also try adding a pinch of Himalayan salt to your water, which can help to replenish electrolytes lost during fasting. Additionally, consuming hydrating foods such as fruits and vegetables can also contribute to maintaining proper hydration levels.

5 Tips To Start IF

IDENTIFY PERSONAL GOALS

Having a personal reason for choosing IF can help you stay motivated and committed to the process. Some common reasons for choosing IF include weight loss, improving insulin sensitivity, reducing inflammation, and increasing longevity. It's important to identify your specific reason for choosing IF and keep it in mind throughout your fasting journey. This can help you overcome any challenges or setbacks and ultimately achieve your goals.

FIGURE OUT YOUR IF PLAN

Figuring out your IF plan is crucial to ensuring your success with intermittent fasting. It is important to choose a plan that suits your lifestyle, eating habits, and health goals. For example, if you are new to fasting, starting with a 12-hour fasting window and gradually increasing it over time can help your body adapt easily to the changes, and you will face minimal side effects. Additionally, it is important to be flexible with your plan and make adjustments as necessary to ensure it works for you. Consistency is key, and sticking to a plan that works for you will help you achieve your health goals with IF.

FIGURE OUT YOUR CALORIE NEEDS

It is important to determine your calorie needs before starting an intermittent fasting plan. While there are no strict diet plans, it is crucial to ensure that whatever you are eating during your eating window is contributing to a net calorie deficit. This means that the total number of calories you consume during your eating window should be lower than the number of calories you burn during the fasting period.

To figure out your calorie needs, you can use an online calculator or consult with a registered dietitian. Your calorie needs may vary based on your age, gender, weight, height, activity level, and other factors. Once you have determined your calorie needs, you can plan your meals accordingly to ensure that you are eating a healthy and balanced diet during your eating window.

FIGURE OUT YOUR MEAL PLAN

meal planning ahead of initiating a fasting program can be very helpful. When you plan your meals ahead of time, you have the opportunity to incorporate a variety of nutritious foods that can help you meet your nutritional needs while you are fasting. This can be particularly important if you are new to fasting or have specific dietary needs or restrictions. Planning your meals can also help you avoid unhealthy food choices that might derail your fasting program. Additionally, meal planning can save time and money by helping you make more efficient use of the foods you have on hand and reducing the need for frequent trips to the grocery store.

OPTIMIZE THE EFFECTS OF IF

While flexibility is an advantage of IF, it's important to maintain a consistent routine to avoid confusion and disruptions in the body's circadian rhythm. It's recommended to establish a regular fasting schedule and stick to it as closely as possible. That being said, there may be some room for adjusting the fasting window or changing up the types of foods consumed during the eating window to maintain variety and prevent boredom or monotony. However, any major changes to the fasting schedule should be made gradually to allow the body to adjust and avoid any adverse effects.

Fasting Tips for women over 50

Here are some intermittent fasting tips for women over 50:

Consult with your healthcare professional before starting an intermittent fasting program.

Start with a more relaxed approach, such as a 12:12 or 14:10 fast, and gradually increase the fasting window.

Stay hydrated by drinking plenty of water during the fasting window.

Focus on nutrient-dense foods during the eating window, including lean proteins, healthy fats, and fiber-rich fruits and vegetables.

Incorporate resistance training or weight-bearing exercises to help maintain muscle mass, which can decrease with age.

Be mindful of portion sizes during the eating window to ensure that you are not overeating.

Listen to your body and adjust your fasting schedule as needed to avoid any adverse effects.

Consider supplementing with vitamins and minerals, as nutrient absorption can decrease with age.

Get adequate sleep and manage stress levels, as these can affect hormone regulation and overall health.

If you experience any negative side effects, such as dizziness, headaches, or fatigue, consult with your healthcare professional and consider adjusting your fasting schedule or approach.

Chapter 3
The Meal Plans and Shopping Lists

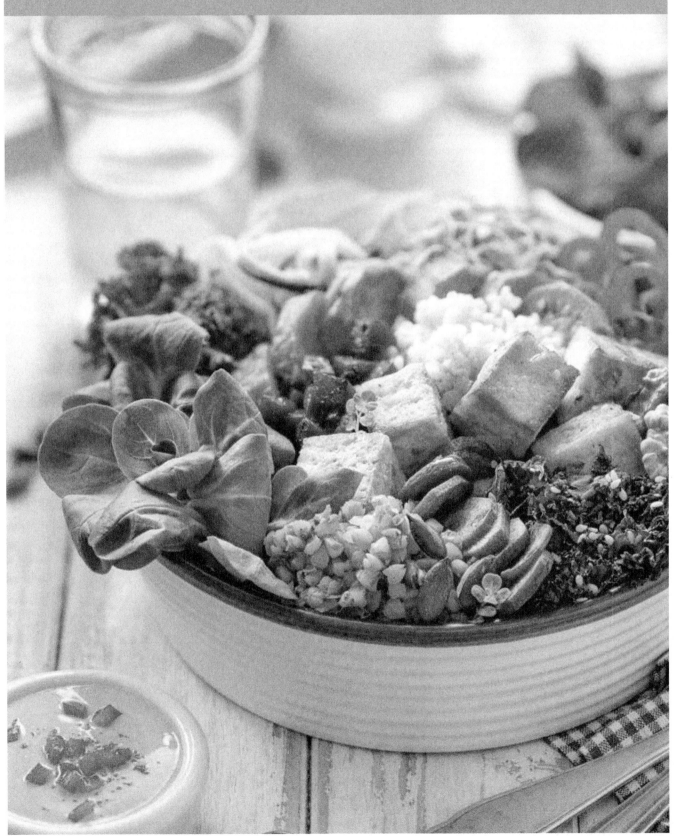

The Conventional Menus: Week 1

Day 1

Meal 1: Banana & Apple Blend
Snack 1: Honey Panna Cotta
Meal 2: Tasty Thai Broth
Snack 2: Honey Panna Cotta

Day 2

Meal 1: Banana & Apple Blend
Snack 1: Honey Panna Cotta
Meal 2: Tasty Thai Broth
Snack 2: Honey Panna Cotta

Day 3

Meal 1: Sympton Soothing Smoothie
Snack 1: Honey Panna Cotta
Meal 2: Tomato & Olive Chicken Fiesta
Snack 2: Honey Panna Cotta

Day 4

Meal 1: Sympton Soothing Smoothie
Snack 1: French Meringues
Meal 2: Tomato & Olive Chicken Fiesta
Snack 2: French Meringues

Day 5

Meal 1: Blackberry & Ginger Milkshake
Snack 1: French Meringues
Meal 2: Seared Ahi Tuna
Snack 2: French Meringues

Day 6

Meal 1: Blackberry & Ginger Milkshake
Snack 1: French Meringues
Meal 2: Seared Ahi Tuna
Snack 2: French Meringues

Day 7

Meal 1: Blackberry & Ginger Milkshake
Snack 1: French Meringues
Meal 2: Seared Ahi Tuna
Snack 2: French Meringues

Shopping List for Week 1

Proteins
2 skinless cod pieces
2 free range skinless chicken breasts
1-lb [455-g] ahi tuna fillet
4 large eggs

Vegetables

3 cups of spinach
1 stalk celery
1 cup cucumber
Ginger
1 white onion
red chili
2 cans chopped tomatoes
1 vanilla bean

Fruits
Banana
4 Apples
Pineapple
Lemon
2 cups blackberries
2 cups chopped peaches
honey

Miscellaneous
flaxseed oil
2 tbsp whole oat bran
1 cup low fat coconut milk
almond milk
chicken broth

Nuts
cilantro seeds

The Conventional Menus: Week 2

Day 1

Meal 1: Almond & Turmeric Chai Tea
Snack 1: French Meringues
Meal 2: Mississippi Pot Roast
Snack 2: French Meringues

Day 2

Meal 1: Almond & Turmeric Chai Tea
Snack 1: Mini Mocha Bundt Cakes
Meal 2: Mississippi Pot Roast
Snack 2: Mini Mocha Bundt Cakes

Day 3

Meal 1: Almond & Turmeric Chai Tea
Snack 1: Mini Mocha Bundt Cakes
Meal 2: Mississippi Pot Roast
Snack 2: Mini Mocha Bundt Cakes

Day 4

Meal 1: Almond & Turmeric Chai Tea
Snack 1: Mini Mocha Bundt Cakes
Meal 2: Mississippi Pot Roast
Snack 2: Mini Mocha Bundt Cakes

Day 5

Meal 1: Orange and Banana Drink

Snack 1: Mini Mocha Bundt Cakes
Meal 2: Mississippi Pot Roast
Snack 2: Mini Mocha Bundt Cakes

Day 6

Meal 1: Orange and Banana Drink
Snack 1: Mini Mocha Bundt Cakes
Meal 2: Chicken Chile Verde
Snack 2: Mini Mocha Bundt Cakes

Day 7

Meal 1: Blueberry Smoothie
Snack 1: Mini Mocha Bundt Cakes
Meal 2: Chicken Chile Verde
Snack 2: Mini Mocha Bundt Cakes

Shopping List for Week 2

Proteins
8 bone-in, skin-on chicken thighs
12 eggs

Vegetables
Ginger
1 tsp cayenne pepper
1½ cups grated zucchini

Fruits
½ cup blueberries
Banana
3 oranges

Miscellaneous
3 tbsp turmeric
4 tsp cinnamon
1/8 tsp ground cloves
1 tsp ground cardamom
Honey
almond milk
8 tablespoons butter
chicken or vegetable stock
3 cups blanched almond flour

Nuts
½ cup chopped walnuts or pecans

The Conventional Menus: Week 3

Day 1

Meal 1: Zucchini Muffins
Snack 1: Mint Chocolate Whoopie Pies
Meal 2: Chicken Pho
Snack 2: Cheesecake Fat Bombs

Day 2

Meal 1: Zucchini Muffins

Snack 1: Mint Chocolate Whoopie Pies
Meal 2: Chicken Pho
Snack 2: Cheesecake Fat Bombs

Day 3

Meal 1: Zucchini Muffins
Snack 1: Mint Chocolate Whoopie Pies
Meal 2: Chicken Pho
Snack 2: Cheesecake Fat Bombs

Day 4

Meal 1: Zucchini Muffins
Snack 1: Mint Chocolate Whoopie Pies
Meal 2: Chicken Pho
Snack 2: Cheesecake Fat Bombs

Day 5

Meal 1: Homemade Apple Tea
Snack 1: Mint Chocolate Whoopie Pies
Meal 2: Lamb Burgers
Snack 2: Cheesecake Fat Bombs

Day 6

Meal 1: Homemade Apple Tea
Snack 1: Mint Chocolate Whoopie Pies
Meal 2: Lamb Burgers
Snack 2: Cheesecake Fat Bombs

Day 7

Meal 1: Homemade Apple Tea
Snack 1: Cheesecake Fat Bombs
Meal 2: Lamb Burgers
Snack 2: Cheesecake Fat Bombs

Shopping List for Week 3

Proteins
4- to 5-lb [1.8- to 2.3-kg] chicken
1 lb [455 g] ground lamb
8 oz [230 g] ground pork
3 large eggs

Vegetables
2 small grated zucchinis
2 yellow onions
fresh ginger
2 jalapeños

Fruits
5 bananas
5 apples

Miscellaneous
walnut butter
coconut milk
fresh green tea leaves

cinnamon
1 lb [455 g] dried brown rice noodles
1 cup [230 g] Greek yogurt
almond flour
¼ cup heavy cream
unsalted butter

The Conventional Menus: Week 4

Day 1

Meal 1: Fresh Cranberry And Lime Juice
Snack 1: Iced Gingerbread Cookies
Meal 2: Smoked Salmon Hash Browns
Snack 2: Iced Gingerbread Cookies

Day 2

Meal 1: Fresh Cranberry And Lime Juice
Snack 1: Iced Gingerbread Cookies
Meal 2: Smoked Salmon Hash Browns
Snack 2: Iced Gingerbread Cookies

Day 3

Meal 1: Fresh Cranberry And Lime Juice
Snack 1: Iced Gingerbread Cookies
Meal 2: Smoked Salmon Hash Browns
Snack 2: Iced Gingerbread Cookies

Day 4

Meal 1: Fresh Cranberry And Lime Juice
Snack 1: Iced Gingerbread Cookies
Meal 2: Smoked Salmon Hash Browns
Snack 2: Iced Gingerbread Cookies

Day 5

Meal 1: Hemp Seed Porridge
Snack 1: Malted Milk Ball Cheesecake
Meal 2: Terrific Turkey Burgers
Snack 2: Malted Milk Ball Cheesecake

Day 6

Meal 1: Hemp Seed Porridge
Snack 1: Malted Milk Ball Cheesecake
Meal 2: Terrific Turkey Burgers
Snack 2: Malted Milk Ball Cheesecake

Day 7

Meal 1: Hemp Seed Porridge
Snack 1: Malted Milk Ball Cheesecake
Meal 2: Terrific Turkey Burgers
Snack 2: Malted Milk Ball Cheesecake

Shopping List for Week 4

Proteins
1 pack smoked salmon

8 oz lean ground turkey meat
3 large eggs

Vegetables
spinach
1 large sweet potato
1 leek
2 cups dill
1 white onion
1 carrot
2 celery stalks
1 red bell pepper
Ginger

Fruits
4 cups cranberries
2 limes
1 cup of mixed berries

Miscellaneous
unsalted butter
1 teaspoon vanilla extract
4 tablespoons ground cinnamon
almond flour
heavy (whipping) cream
coconut milk

Nuts
3 cups cooked hemp seed

Chapter 4
Smoothies And Drinks

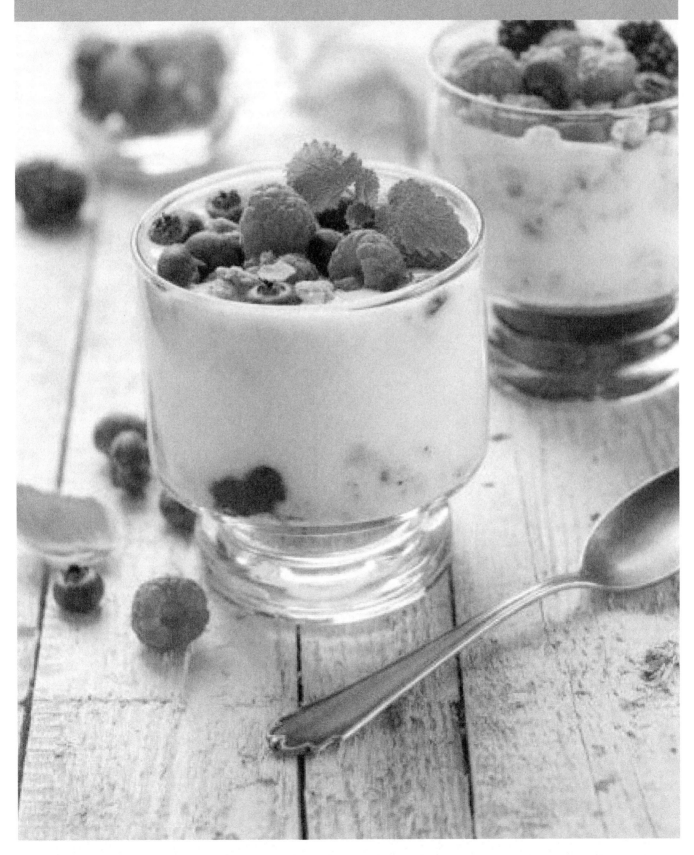

Gingery Green Iced-Tea

Prep time: 2 minutes|Cook time:0 minutes|Serves 1

- 2 cups concentrated green or
- macha tea, served hot
- 1/4 cup crystalized ginger, chopped into fine pieces
- 1 sprig of fresh mint

1. Get a glass container and mix the tea with the ginger and then cover and chill for as long as time permits.
2. Strain and pour into serving glasses over ice if you wish.
3. Garnish with a wedge of lemon and a sprig of fresh mint to serve.

Banana & Apple Blend

Prep time: 5 minutes|Cook time:4 minutes|Serves 1

- 1 banana
- 1 apple, cored and peeled
- 2 tbsp flaxseed oil
- 2 tbsp whole oat bran
- 2 cups filtered water
- 1 tbsp stevia
- 1 cup low fat coconut milk
- 1 cup of spinach or equivalent green of your choice

1. In a food processor, add all of the ingredients except for the greens, processing until smooth.
2. Mix in the greens and then blend until smooth.
3. Serve over ice.

Blueberry And Spinach Shake

Prep time: 2 minutes|Cook time:0 minutes|Serves 1

- 1 cup frozen blueberries
- 1/2 banana
- 1/2 cup cucumber, chopped
- 1 tbsp flaxseeds
- 1 cup coconut water

1. Take all of the ingredients and blend until smooth.
2. You can add ice cubes at this point if you want it chilled.
3. Serve.

Sympton Soothing Smoothie

Prep time: 2 minutes|Cook time:0 minutes|Serves 1

- 1 stalk celery, chopped
- 1 cup cucumber, chopped
- 1/2 cup pineapple, chopped
- 1/2 lemon, zest juice
- 1 cup coconut water
- 1 apple, chopped

1. Take all of the ingredients (minus the lemon zest) and blend until smooth.
2. You can add ice cubes at this point if you want it chilled.
3. Serve with a sprinkling of lemon zest.

Wonderful Watermelon Drink
Prep time: 2 minutes|Cook time:0 minutes|Serves 1

- 1 cup watermelon chunks
- 2 cups frozen mixed berries
- 1 cup coconut water
- 2 tbsp chia seeds
- 1/2 cup of tart cherries

1. Blend ingredients in a blender or juicer until pureed.
2. Serve immediately and enjoy!

Almond & Turmeric Chai Tea
Prep time: 2 minutes|Cook time:2 minutes|Serves 4

- 3 tbsp turmeric
- 4 tsp cinnamon
- 1/8 tsp ground cloves
- 1 tsp ground cardamom
- 1 tsp ground ginger
- 1 tsp cayenne pepper
- 4 tsp chai tea powder
- 4 cups boiling water
- honey to taste
- 1 cup almond milk

1. Combine all of the ingredients excluding the milk and honey in a glass container, mix well and then seal.
2. Pour boiling water into 2 tbsp of the tea mix (use a tea strainer to serve).
3. You can then add almond milk and honey to taste.
4. Save the tea mix in a sealed container, storing in a dry place for future chais!

Homemade Apple Tea
Prep time: overnight|Cook time:0 minutes|Serves 4

- 4 cups boiling water
- 4 tbsp fresh green tea leaves
- 5 apples, peeled and sliced.
- 1 tsp cinnamon

1. Pour boiling water over tea leaves through a tea strainer, allowing to steep for 5 minutes.
2. Add the apple slices and cinnamon to the boiling water and transfer into a sealable container.
3. Chill overnight to allow apple to infuse before serving.
4. Garnish with fresh apple slices and mint to serve over ice.

Fresh Cranberry And Lime Juice
Prep time: 5 minutes|Cook time:0 minutes|Serves 4

- 4 cups cranberries
- 2 limes, juiced
- 1/2 cup spinach
- 1/2 cup of mixed berries (frozen are fine)

1. Mix all the ingredients with water in a juicer until pureed and served immediately over ice.

Blackberry & Ginger Milkshake

Prep time: 2 minutes|Cook time:0 minutes|Serves 1

- 1 thumb sized piece of ginger, grated
- 2 cups blackberries, washed
- 2 cups chopped peaches
- 2 cups almond milk

1. Add all the ingredients to a blender or juicer and blend together until smooth.
2. Serve with a scattering of fresh blackberries and enjoy!

Fresh Tropical Juice

Prep time: 5 minutes|Cook time:30 minutes|Serves 4

- 1 whole fresh pineapple, peeled and cut into chunks.
- 1/2 can low fat coconut milk
- 1 cup water

1. Add all ingredients to a juicer and blend until smooth.
2. Serve over ice.

Orange and Banana Drink

Prep time: 5 minutes|Cook time:0 minutes|Serves 2

- ½ of a burro banana, peeled
- 3 oranges, peeled
- 1½ tablespoons Date sugar
- ½ teaspoon Bromide Plus Powder
- 1 cup of soft-jelly coconut water

1. Plug in a high-speed food processor or blender and add all the ingredients in its jar.
2. Cover the blender jar with its lid and then pulse for 40 to 60 seconds until smooth.
3. Divide the drink between two glasses and then serve.

Dandelion Revitalizing Smoothie

Prep time: 5 minutes|Cook time:0 minutes|Serves 2

- ¼ cup blueberries
- ½ of a large bunch of dandelion greens
- 2 baby burro bananas, peeled
- ½ cup watercress
- 3 dates, pitted
- 1 tablespoon Bromide Plus powder
- 1 cup of soft-jelly coconut water
- 2 tablespoons lime juice

1. Plug in a high-speed food processor or blender and add all the ingredients in its jar.
2. Cover the blender jar with its lid and then pulse for 40 to 60 seconds until smooth. Divide the drink between two glasses and then serve.

Amazing Sea Moss Green Drink

Prep time: 5 minutes|Cook time:0 minutes|Serves 2

- 4 tablespoons of sea moss gel
- 4 cups mixed greens
- 2 burro banana, peeled

1. Plug in a high-speed food processor or blender and add all the ingredients in its jar.
2. Cover the blender jar with its lid and then pulse for 40 to 60 seconds until smooth.
3. Divide the drink between two glasses and then serve.

Blueberry-Pie Smoothie

Prep time: 5 minutes|Cook time:0 minutes|Serves 1

- ¼ cup cooked amaranth
- 1 cup blueberries
- 1 teaspoon Bromide Plus Powder
- 1 burro banana, peeled
- 1 tablespoon walnut butter, homemade (Optional)
- 2 tablespoons date sugar
- 1 cup soft-jelly coconut milk, homemade

1. Plug in a high-speed food processor or blender and add all the ingredients in its jar.
2. Cover the blender jar with its lid and then pulse for 40 to 60 seconds until smooth.
3. Divide the drink between two glasses and then serve.

Mixed Fruit & Nut Milkshake

Prep time: 5 minutes|Cook time:30 minutes|Serves 4

- 1/2½ grapefruit, peeled and chopped
- 2 tbsp chopped almonds
- 1/2½ inch piece of ginger, minced
- juice of 1 orange
- 1 tbsp honey
- 1/2 cup almond milk
- 12 strawberries

1. Put everything but the strawberries in a blender until smooth.
2. Add in the strawberries and blend until pureed, serving in a tall glass.

Blueberry Smoothie

Prep time: 5 minutes|Cook time:0 minutes|Serves 2

- ½ cup blueberries
- 1 burro banana, peeled
- 2 tablespoon date sugar (Optional)
- 1 cup Hemp milk, homemade (Optional)

1. Plug in a high-speed food processor or blender and add all the ingredients in its jar.
2. Cover the blender jar with its lid and then pulse for 40 to 60 seconds until smooth.
3. Divide the drink between two glasses and then serve.

Green Smoothie with Sea Moss

Prep time: 5 minutes|Cook time:10 minutes|Serves 2

- 1 cup raspberries
- 1 cup kale leaves
- 1 tablespoon sea moss
- 2 tablespoons key lime juice
- 1 cup soft-jelly coconut milk

1. Plug in a high-speed food processor or blender and add all the ingredients in its jar.
2. Cover the blender jar with its lid and then pulse for 40 to 60 seconds until smooth.
3. Divide the drink between two glasses and then serve.

Papaya and Amaranth Smoothie

Prep time: 5 minutes|Cook time:10 minutes|Serves 2

- 2 cups papaya cubes
- 2 tablespoons date sugar
- 1 cup cooked amaranth
- 2 teaspoons Bromide Plus Powder
- 2 cups hemp milk, homemade

1. Plug in a high-speed food processor or blender and add all the ingredients in its jar.
2. Cover the blender jar with its lid and then pulse for 40 to 60 seconds until smooth.
3. Divide the drink between two glasses and then serve.

Lettuce, Banana and Berries Smoothie

Prep time: 5 minutes|Cook time:0 minutes|Serves 2

- ½ of a burro banana
- ¼ cup blueberries
- 1 cup Romaine lettuce
- 2 tablespoons key lime juice
- ½ cup soft jelly coconut water

1. Plug in a high-speed food processor or blender and add all the ingredients in its jar.
2. Cover the blender jar with its lid and then pulse for 40 to 60 seconds until smooth.
3. Divide the drink between two glasses and then serve.

Green Sea Moss Drink

Prep time: 5 minutes|Cook time:0 minutes|Serves 2

- 1 apple, cored, diced
- 2 cups kale
- 1 cup cucumber chunks
- 2 cups of coconut water
- 1 key lime, juiced
- 1 tablespoon of sea moss gel

1. Plug in a high-speed food processor or blender and add all the ingredients in its jar.
2. Cover the blender jar with its lid and then pulse for 40 to 60 seconds until smooth.
3. Divide the drink between two glasses and then serve.

Veggie-Ful Smoothie

Prep time: 5 minutes|Cook time:0 minutes|Serves 2

- 1 pear, cored, deseeded
- ½ cup watercress
- ¼ of avocado, peeled
- ½ cup Romaine lettuce
- ½ of cucumber, peeled, deseeded
- 1 tablespoon date sugar
- ½ cup spring water

1. Plug in a high-speed food processor or blender and add all the ingredients in its jar.
2. Cover the blender jar with its lid and then pulse for 40 to 60 seconds until smooth.
3. Divide the drink between two glasses and then serve.

Chapter 5
Breakfast

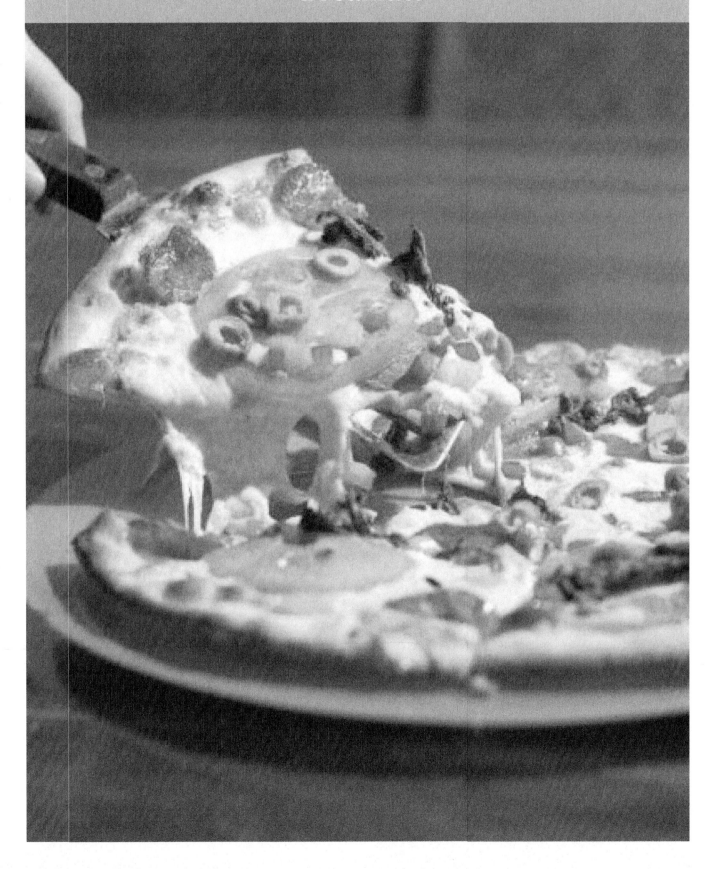

Alkaline Blueberry Spelt Pancakes

Prep time: 6 minutes|Cook time:20 minutes|Serves 3

- 2 cups spelt flour
- 1 cup coconut milk
- 1/2 cup alkaline water
- 2 tbsps. grapeseed oil
- 1/2 cup agave
- 1/2 cup blueberries
- 1/4 tsp. sea moss

1. Mix the spelled flour, agave, grapeseed oil, hemp seeds, and sea moss together in a bowl.
2. Add 1 cup of hemp milk and alkaline water to the mixture until you get the consistent mixture you like.
3. Crimp the blueberries into the batter.
4. Heat the skillet to moderate heat, then lightly coat it with the grapeseed oil.
5. Pour the batter into the skillet and let them cook for approximately 5 minutes on every side.
6. Serve and Enjoy.

Alkaline Blueberry Muffins

Prep time: 5 minutes|Cook time:20 minutes|Serves 3

- 1 cup coconut milk
- 3/4 cup spelt flour
- 3/4 tef flour
- 1/2 cup blueberries
- 1/3 cup agave
- 1/4 cup sea moss gel
- 1/2 tsp. sea salt
- Grapeseed oil

1. Adjust the temperature of the oven to 365 degrees.
2. Grease 6 regular-size muffin cups with muffin liners.
3. In a bowl, mix together sea salt, sea moss, agave, coconut milk, and flour gel until properly blended.
4. You then crimp in blueberries.
5. Coat the muffin pan lightly with the grapeseed oil.
6. Pour in the muffin batter.
7. Bake for at least 30 minutes until it turns golden brown.
8. Serve.

Crunchy Quinoa Meal

Prep time: 5 minutes|Cook time:25 minutes|Serves 2

- 3 cups coconut milk
- 1 cup rinsed quinoa
- 1 cup raspberry
- 1/2 cup chopped coconut

1. In a saucepan, pour milk and boil over moderate heat.
2. Add the quinoa to the milk, and then bring it to a boil once more.
3. You then let it simmer for at least 15 minutes on medium heat until the milk is reduced.
4. Cover it and cook for 8 minutes until the milk is completely absorbed.
5. Add the raspberry and cook the meal for 30 seconds.
6. Serve and enjoy.

Zucchini Muffins

Prep time: 10 minutes|Cook time:25 minutes|Serves 16

- 1 tbsp. ground flaxseed
- 3 tbsps. spring water
- 1/4 cup walnut butter
- 3 medium over-ripe bananas
- 2 small grated zucchinis
- 1/2 cup coconut milk
- 2 cups coconut flour
- 1/4 tsp. sea salt

1. Adjust the temperature of your oven to 375°F.
2. Grease the muffin tray with the cooking spray.
3. In a bowl, mix the flaxseed with water.
4. In a glass bowl, mash the bananas, then stir in the remaining ingredients.
5. Properly mix and then divide the mixture into the muffin tray.
6. Bake it for 25 minutes.
7. Serve.

Hemp Seed Porridge

Prep time: 5 minutes|Cook time:5 minutes|Serves 6

- 3 cups cooked hemp seed
- 1 cup coconut milk

1. In a saucepan, mix the rice and the coconut milk over moderate heat for about 5 minutes as you stir it constantly.
2. Remove the pan from the heat, then stir.
3. Serve in 6 bowls.
4. Enjoy.

Banana Barley Porridge

Prep time: 15 minutes|Cook time:5 minutes|Serves 2

- 1 cup divided unsweetened coconut milk
- 1 small peeled and sliced banana
- 1/2 cup barley
- 1/4 cup chopped coconuts

1. In a bowl, properly mix barley with half of the coconut milk.
2. Cover the bowl, then refrigerate for about 6 hours.
3. In a saucepan, mix the barley mixture with coconut milk.
4. Cook for about 5 minutes on moderate heat.
5. Then top it with the chopped coconuts and the banana slices.
6. Serve.

Coconut Pancakes

Prep time: 5 minutes|Cook time:15 minutes|Serves 4

- 1 cup coconut flour
- 2 tbsps. arrowroot powder
- 1 tsp. baking powder
- 1 cup coconut milk
- 3 tbsps. coconut oil

1. In a medium container, mix in all the dry ingredients.
2. Add the coconut milk and 2 tbsps. Of the coconut oil, then mix properly.
3. In a skillet, melt 1 tsp of coconut oil.
4. Pour a ladle of the batter into the skillet, then swirl the pan to spread the batter evenly into a smooth pancake.
5. Cook it for at least 3 minutes on medium heat until it becomes firm.
6. Turn the pancake to the other side and cook it for another 2 minutes until it turns golden brown.
7. Cook the remaining pancakes in the same process.
8. Serve.

Alkaline Blueberry and Strawberry Muffins

Prep time: 15 minutes|Cook time:5 hours|Serves 6

- 3/4 cup quinoa flour
- 3/4 cup tef flour
- 1/2 teaspoon salt
- 1/3 cup agave
- 1 cup fresh coconut milk
- 1/4 cup strawberries, chopped
- 1/4 cup blueberries

1. Place the quinoa flour, tef flour, and salt in a bowl.
2. In another bowl, combine the agave and coconut milk. Slowly pour the wet ingredients into the dry ingredients.
3. Mix until well-combined.
4. Stir in the berries and mix until well-combined.
5. Pour the batter into muffin pans.
6. Place the muffin pans with the batter in the Instant Pot.
7. Close the lid but do not set the vent to the Sealing position.
8. Press the Slow Cook button and adjust the cooking time to 4 to 5 hours.

Blueberry Spelt Flat Cakes

Prep time: 15 minutes|Cook time:4 hours|Serves 4

- 2 cups spelt flour
- 1/4 teaspoon sea salt
- 1/4 cup hemp seeds
- 1 cup fresh coconut milk
- 1/2 cup spring water
- 2 tablespoons grapeseed oil
- 1/2 cup agave
- 1/2 cup blueberries

1. Mix the spelt flour, sea salt, and hemp seeds in a bowl.
2. Pour in the coconut milk, water, grapeseed oil, and agave.
3. Stir until well-combined. Pour in the blueberries.
4. Line the Instant Pot with parchment paper.
5. Pour the batter into the Instant Pot.
6. Close the lid but do not set the vent to the Sealing position.
7. Press the Slow Cook button and adjust the cooking time to 4 hours.

Breakfast Quinoa Cereal

Prep time: 15 minutes|Cook time:15 minutes|Serves 2

- 1 cup quinoa
- 2 cups spring water
- A dash of cayenne pepper
- A dash of sea salt
- A dash of oregano

1. Place the quinoa and spring water in the Instant Pot. Give a good stir.
2. Close the lid and set the vent to the Sealing position.
3. Press the Multigrain button and adjust the cooking time to 15 minutes.
4. Do natural pressures release.
5. Once the lid is open, ladle the porridge in bowls and top with cayenne pepper, salt, and oregano.

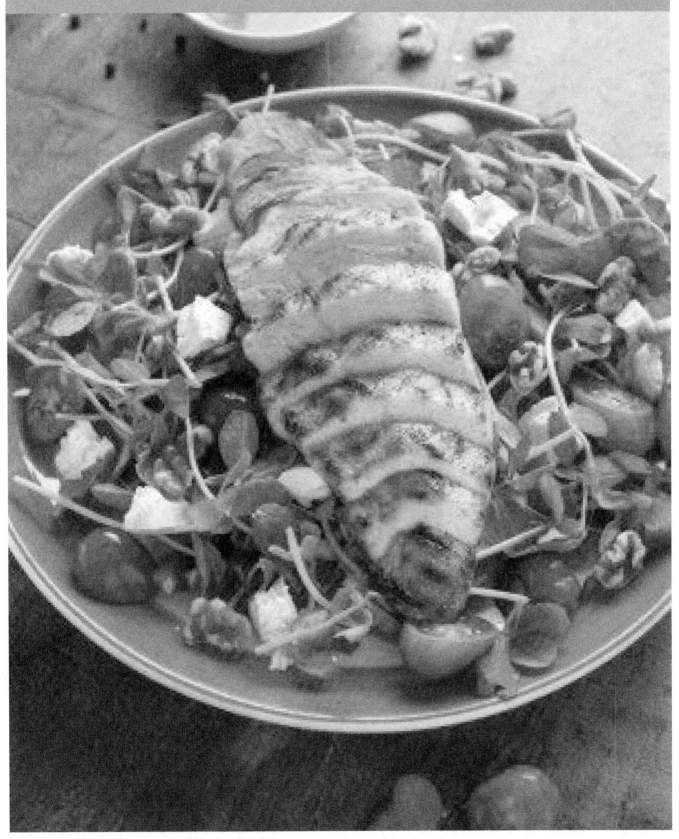

Tomato & Olive Chicken Fiesta

Prep time: 5 minutes|Cook time:35 minutes|Serves 2

- 2 free range skinless chicken breasts
- 1 onion, roughly chopped
- 2 garlic cloves, chopped
- 2 cans chopped tomatoes
- 1 tbsp balsamic vinegar
- 8 green olives, chopped
- 2 cups homemade chicken stock
- handful of fresh basil leaves
- a pinch of black pepper

1. Preheat oven to 375°F/190 °C/Gas Mark 5.
2. Add the onion, garlic, chopped tomatoes, olives, chicken stock and balsamic vinegar to the pan with most of the basil leaves and cover.
3. Place in the oven for 35-40 minutes or until chicken is cooked throughout.
4. Plate up and serve with the remaining basil as a garnish.

Cajun Chicken & Prawn

Prep time: 5 minutes|Cook time:35 minutes|Serves 2

- 2 free range skinless chicken breasts, chopped
- 1 onion, chopped
- 1 red pepper, chopped
- 2 garlic cloves, crushed
- 10 fresh or frozen king prawns
- 1 tsp cayenne pepper
- 1 tsp chili powder
- 1 tsp paprika
- 1/4 tsp chili powder
- 1 tsp dried oregano
- 1 tsp dried thyme
- 1 cup brown or wholegrain rice
- 1 tbsp extra virgin olive oil
- 1 can chopped tomatoes
- 2 cups homemade chicken stock

1. Mix the spices and herbs in a separate bowl to form your Cajun spice mix.
2. Grab a large pan and add the olive oil, heating on a medium heat.
3. Add the chicken and brown each side for around 4-5 minutes. Place to one side.
4. Add the onion to the pan and fry until soft.
5. Add the garlic, prawns, Cajun seasoning and red pepper to the pan and cook for around 5 minutes or until prawns become opaque.
6. Add the brown rice along with the chopped tomatoes, chicken and chicken stock to the pan.
7. Cover the pan and allow to simmer for around 25 minutes or until the rice is soft.
8. Serve and enjoy!

Harissa Spiced Chicken Tray-Bake
Prep time: 10 minutes|Cook time:25 minutes|Serves 4

- 4 free range skinless chicken breasts, diced
- 1/2 cup of low-fat greek yogurt
- 1 small butternut squash, chopped
- and peeled
- 2 red onions, chopped
- for the harissa paste:
- 1 red pepper, diced
- 1 tsp dried red chilli,
- 1 garlic clove, minced
- 1 tsp caraway seeds, crushed
- 1 tsp ground cumin
- 1 tsp fresh or dried coriander,
- 1 tbsp tomato purée (no added salt or sugar)
- 1 tbsp extra virgin olive oil

1. Pre-heat oven to 375°F/190 °C/Gas Mark 5.
2. In a bowl, combine the ingredients for the harissa paste and then add 3 tbsp yogurt.
3. Coat the chicken breasts with the mixture, cover and leave to one side.
4. Scatter the chicken pieces, onions and chopped butternut squash with the harissa paste over a baking tray and place in the oven for 35 minutes or until the chicken is cooked right through.
5. Plate up and serve with the remaining yogurt.

Terrific Turkey Burgers
Prep time: 5 minutes|Cook time:35 minutes|Serves 6

- 8 oz lean ground turkey meat
- 1 white onions, minced
- 1 carrot, shredded
- 2 celery stalks, finely chopped
- 1 red bell pepper, finely chopped (optional)
- 1 tbsp dill
- 1 tsp cilantro
- 1 tsp dry mustard
- 2 tbsp olive oil
- pinch of black pepper to taste

1. Pre-heat oven to 390°F/200 °C/Gas Mark 6.
2. Add the vegetables in a bowl with the olive oil, pepper and herbs and then mix well.
3. Add in the meat and mix with wet hands to create two patties.
4. Place the patties on a lightly oiled baking tray and bake in the oven for 25-30 minutes or until meat is cooked through (flip half way).
5. Turn up the broiler and broil for the last 5 minutes for a golden and crispy edge.
6. Serve on a bed of your favorite salad.

Super Sesame Chicken Noodles

Prep time: 10 minutes|Cook time:20 minutes|Serves 2

- 2 free range skinless chicken breasts, chopped
- 1 cup rice/buckwheat noodles such as japanese udon
- 1 carrot, chopped
- 1/2 orange, juiced
- 1 tsp sesame seeds
- 2 tsp coconut oil
- 1 thumb sized piece of ginger, minced
- 1/2 cup sugar snap peas

1. Heat 1 tsp oil on a medium heat in a skillet.
2. Sauté the chopped chicken breast for about 10-15 minutes or until cooked through.
3. While cooking the chicken, place the noodles, carrots and peas in a pot of boiling water for about 5 minutes. Drain.
4. In a bowl, mix together the ginger, sesame seeds, 1 tsp oil and orange juice to make your dressing.
5. Once chicken is cooked and noodles are cooked and drained, add the chicken, noodles, carrots and peas to the dressing and toss.
6. Serve warm or chilled.

Lebanese Chicken Kebabs And Hummus

Prep time: 10 minutes|Cook time:25 minutes|Serves 4

- for the chicken:
- 1 cup lemon juice
- 8 garlic cloves, minced
- 1 tbsp thyme, finely chopped
- 1 tbsp paprika
- 2 tsp ground cumin
- 1 tsp cayenne pepper
- 4 free range skinless chicken
- breasts, cubed
- 4 metal kebab skewers
- lemon wedges to garnish
- for the hummus:
- 1 can chickpeas/ 1 cup dried
- chickpeas soaked overnight
- 2 tbsp tahini paste
- 1 lemon, juiced
- 1 tsp turmeric
- 1 tsp black pepper
- 2 tbsp olive oil

1. Whisk the lemon juice, garlic, thyme, paprika, cumin, and cayenne pepper in a bowl.
2. Skewer the chicken cubes using kebab sticks (metal).
3. Baste the chicken on each side with the marinade, covering for as long as possible in the fridge (the lemon juice will tenderize the meat and means it will be more suitable for the anti-inflammatory diet).
4. When ready to cook, preheat the oven to 400°F/200 °C/Gas Mark 6 and bake for 20-25 minutes or until chicken is thoroughly cooked through.
5. Prepare the hummus by adding the ingredients to a blender and whizzing up until smooth.
6. If it is a little thick and chunky, add a little water to loosen the mix.
7. Serve the chicken kebabs, garnished with the lemon wedges and the hummus on the side.

Chicken Chile Verde

Prep time: 15 minutes|Cook time:2 hours 15minutes|Serves 4 to 6

- 8 bone-in, skin-on chicken thighs
- Kosher salt
- Freshly ground black pepper
- 2 Tbsp extra-virgin olive oil
- 1/2 cup [120 ml] chicken or vegetable stock
- 2 cups [460 g] Tomatillo and Jalapeño Salsa Verde or other salsa verde

1. In a large sauté pan over medium-high heat, warm the olive oil until just smoking.
2. Working in batches, add the chicken thighs skin-side down and cook until the skin is golden brown and very crispy, 5 to 6 minutes.
3. Turn, cooking the other side for 3 to 4 minutes, then transfer the chicken to a plate.
4. Once all the chicken thighs have been seared, pour off any accumulated fat and return the pan to medium-high heat.
5. Add the chicken stock and salsa verde and bring to a boil, scraping up any browned bits from the bottom of the pan.
6. Pour the mixture into a slow cooker and nestle the chicken thighs on top.
7. Cover and cook until the chicken is fork-tender, about 2 hours on the high setting or about 4 hours on the low setting.
8. Skim any excess fat off the surface before serving.

Country Captain'S Chicken

Prep time: 30 minutes|Cook time:1 hour 10 minutes|Serves 4 to 6

- One 4- to 5-lb [1.8- to 2.3-kg] chicken, cut into 8 pieces
- Kosher salt
- 2 Tbsp extra-virgin olive oil
- 1 large red onion, thinly sliced
- 3 celery stalks, sliced
- 11/2 Tbsp curry powder
- Freshly ground black pepper
- 2 Tbsp tomato paste (optional if nightshade-sensitive)
- One 28-oz [800-g] can diced tomatoes (optional if nightshade-sensitive)
- 1 cup [240 ml] chicken or vegetable stock
- 1/2 cup [85 g] raisins
- 1/2 cup [65 g] raw almonds, toasted and coarsely chopped
- 4 cups [520 g] cooked brown rice
- 2 Tbsp chopped parsley

1. Rinse the chicken pieces and pat dry thoroughly.
2. Season with salt.
3. In a large Dutch oven or stockpot over medium-high heat, warm the olive oil until just smoking.
4. Working in batches, sear the chicken until well browned on both sides, 8 to 10 minutes per batch.
5. Transfer the chicken to a platter and pour off all

but 2 Tbsp of the accumulated fat. (If the bottom of the pot is scorched, discard the oil, wipe it clean, and add another 2 Tbsp oil.)
6. Turn the heat to medium and add the onion and celery.
7. Cook, stirring frequently, until the onion is soft, 5 to 7 minutes.
8. Add the curry powder, 1/2 tsp black pepper, and tomato paste (if using) and cook, stirring constantly, until fragrant, about 30 seconds.
9. Add the tomatoes with their juices (if using), chicken stock, and raisins and bring to a simmer, scraping the bottom of the pot to remove all the caramelized bits.
10. Nestle the chicken into the pot, cover, and turn the heat to medium-low.
11. Simmer until chicken thighs are fork-tender, about 45 minutes.
12. Transfer the chicken to a platter, turn the heat to medium-high, and cook, stirring occasionally, until the sauce has reduced slightly, 5 to 7 minutes.
13. Taste, adding more salt and pepper if necessary.
14. Stir the toasted almonds into the brown rice.
15. Spoon on plates and top with the chicken and sauce.
16. Finish with the parsley.
17. Serve immediately.
18. make it ahead.
19. Preparing this braise a day or two in advance will only enhance the flavors, making it the ideal dish for company or a wonderful make-ahead meal for a weeknight dinner.
20. Once it cools, store it covered in the refrigerator in the pot you cooked it in.
21. When it's time to reheat, place the covered Dutch oven over low heat.
22. Stir after a few minutes, then cook until the meat is just warmed through, about 10 minutes.

Chicken Pho

Prep time: 30 minutes|Cook time:3 hours|Serves 6

- One 4- to 5-lb [1.8- to 2.3-kg] chicken, quartered, backbone reserved
- 2 yellow onions, peeled and halved
- One 2-in [5-cm] piece fresh ginger, peeled and smashed
- Kosher salt
- 2 tsp light brown sugar
- 5 qt [4.7 L] water
- 1/4 cup [60 ml] fish sauce, plus more for serving
- 1 lb [455 g] dried brown rice noodles, such as Annie Chun's Pad Thai Brown Rice Noodles
- 1 bunch green onions, green parts only, thinly sliced
- 2 cups [120 g] mung bean sprouts
- 2 jalapeños, thinly sliced (optional if nightshade-sensitive)
- Torn basil, cilantro, and mint leaves for serving
- Lime wedges for serving
- Sriracha sauce for serving (optional)

1. Place the chicken pieces and backbone, onions, ginger, 2 tsp salt, brown sugar, and water in a stockpot with at least an 8-qt [7.5-L] capacity.
2. Slowly bring to a boil over medium-high heat. Turn the heat to medium-low and simmer gently, uncovered, for 1 hour, skimming off any impurities that come to the surface. (Add water as necessary to keep the chicken covered.)
3. Using tongs, remove the chicken pieces from the pot and transfer to a cutting board.
4. When the chicken is cool to the touch, remove all the meat from the skin and bones and transfer to a medium bowl.
5. Return the skin and bones to the stockpot.
6. Shred the meat, then cover and refrigerate until ready to serve.
7. Return the stock to a simmer and continue to cook for 11/2 to 2 hours. Using a fine-mesh sieve, strain the stock into another stockpot and cook over high heat until reduced to 12 cups [3 L], about 20 minutes.
8. Stir in the fish sauce. (At this point, you can cool the stock to room temperature, cover, and refrigerate for up to 3 days.)
9. Prepare the rice noodles according to the package instructions.
10. While the noodles cook, add half of the shredded chicken to the stock and simmer until the chicken is warmed through. (Reserve the remaining shredded chicken for another use).
11. Divide the cooked rice noodles among six large soup bowls and sprinkle evenly with the green onions, bean sprouts, and jalapeños (if using).
12. Ladle the stock and chicken over the noodles and finish with the torn herbs.
13. Serve with lime wedges, additional fish sauce, and Sriracha sauce, if desired.
14. a reliable option
15. When shopping in a typical grocery store with a

limited assortment of Asian ingredients, I always turn to Annie Chun's for rice noodles and Thai Kitchen for guaranteed gluten-free fish sauce.

Greek Fennel & Olive Baked Chicken

Prep time: 10 minutes|Cook time:1 hour|Serves 4

- 1 whole free range chicken
- 1 tsp black pepper
- 2 lemons, cut into slices
- 3 cloves garlic, minced
- 1 tbsp oregano, chopped
- 2 tbsp extra virgin olive oil
- 1 fennel bulb, sliced
- 1/3 cup pitted black or kalamata
- olives, halved
- 2 white sweet potatoes, peeled and
- cubed

1. Pre-heat oven to 375°F/190 °C/Gas Mark 5.
2. Pat the chicken dry with kitchen towel and place on a lined baking tray.
3. Use a sharp knife to slide underneath the skin and create a pocket. Sprinkle pepper underneath the skin.
4. Mix 1 tbsp olive oil, lemon zest and juice of the lemons with the garlic and oregano (save the lemon wedges).
5. Pour this into the pocket you created under the skin to marinate for as little or as much time as you have (don't worry if it drizzles out of the pocket).
6. Toss the fennel, sweet potato and olives, 1 tbsp oil and the lemon wedges in a separate bowl.
7. Scatter the fennel mix around the base of the chicken.
8. Bake for 1 hour or following package guidelines to ensure chicken is thoroughly cooked through. Remove the skin and cut into servings of the breasts, legs, thighs and any extra flaky meat you can cut away.
9. Serve immediately with an extra squeeze of lemon juice and some fresh thyme or oregano if desired!

Italian Chicken & Zucchini Spaghetti

Prep time: 10 minutes|Cook time:30 minutes|Serves 2

- for the chicken:
- 2 free range skinless chicken breast, sliced
- 1 tbsp extra virgin olive oil
- juice of 1/2 lemon
- 1 clove garlic, crushed
- 1/2 tsp dried oregano
- pinch of black pepper
- for the pasta:
- 3 zucchinis
- 1 tsp extra virgin olive oil

1. Pre-heat oven to 400°F/200°C/Gas Mark 6.
2. Combine 1 tbsp olive oil, lemon juice, garlic, and oregano and coat the chicken slices.
3. Line a baking sheet with foil or parchment paper.
4. Layer the chicken strips and cook for 25-30 minutes or until cooked through.
5. Meanwhile, prepare your zucchini by slicing into thin spaghetti strips – use a mandolin or spiralyzer and leave in a colander to drain for 10 minutes.
6. When chicken is cooked, remove from the oven and place to one side.
7. Boil a pan of water on a medium heat and add a pinch of black pepper.
8. Add your zucchini spaghetti to the water and boil for one minute before immediately draining.
9. Plate and serve, layering half the chicken on top and drizzling with 1 tsp olive oil and a little black pepper.
10. Enjoy!

Nutty Pesto Chicken Supreme

Prep time: 10 minutes|Cook time:30 minutes|Serves 2

- 2 free range skinless chicken or turkey breasts
- 1 bunch of fresh basil
- 1/2 cup raw spinach
- 1 cup crushed macadamias/
- almonds/walnuts or a combination
- 2 tbsp extra virgin olive oil
- 1/2 cup low fat hard cheese
- (optional)

1. Preheat oven to 350°F/170°C/Gas Mark 4.
2. Take the chicken breasts and use a meat pounder to 'thin' each breast into a 1cm thick escalope.
3. Reserve a handful of the nuts before adding the rest of the ingredients and a little black pepper to a blender or pestle and mortar and blend until smooth (you can leave this a little chunky for a rustic feel if you wish).
4. Add a little water if the pesto needs loosening.
5. Coat the chicken in the pesto.
6. Bake for at least 30 minutes in the oven, or until chicken is completely cooked through.
7. Top each chicken escalope with the remaining nuts and place under the broiler for 5 minutes for a crispy topping to complete.

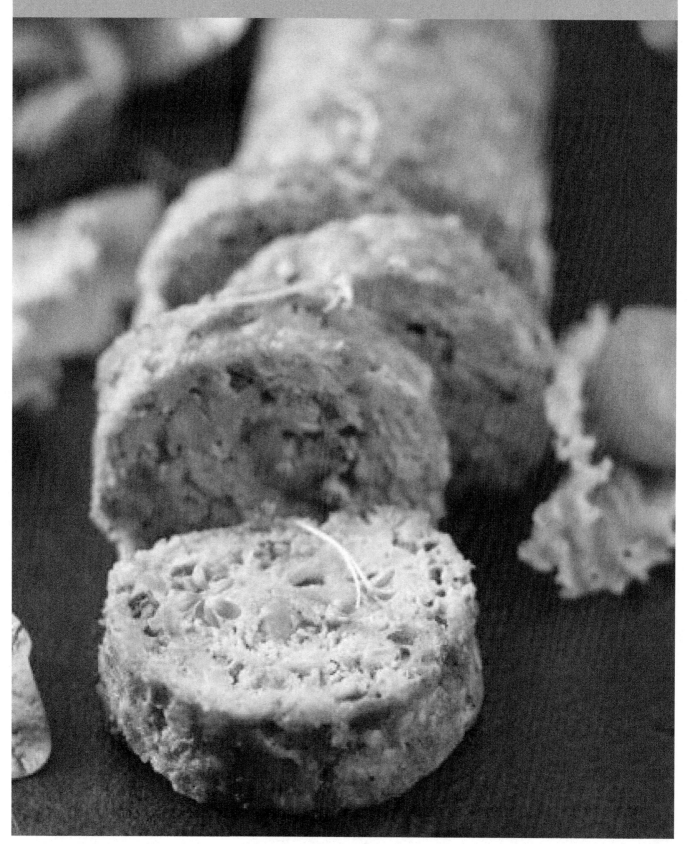

Sesame Pork And Green Beans

Prep time: 5 minutes|Cook time:10 minutes|Serves 2

- Pink Himalayan salt
- Freshly ground black pepper
- 2 tablespoons toasted sesame oil, divided
- 2 tablespoons soy sauce
- 1 teaspoon Sriracha sauce
- 1 cup fresh green beans

1. On a cutting board, pat the pork chops dry with a paper towel.
2. Slice the chops into strips, and season with pink Himalayan salt and pepper.
3. In a large skillet over medium heat, heat 1 tablespoon of sesame oil.
4. Add the pork strips and cook them for 7 minutes, stirring occasionally.
5. In a small bowl, mix to combine the remaining 1 tablespoon of sesame oil, the soy sauce, and the Sriracha sauce.
6. Pour into the skillet with the pork.
7. Add the green beans to the skillet, reduce the heat to medium-low, and simmer for 3 to 5 minutes.
8. Divide the pork, green beans, and sauce between two wide, shallow bowls and serve.

Slow-Cooker Barbecue Ribs

Prep time: 10 minutes|Cook time:4 hours|Serves 2

- Pink Himalayan salt
- Freshly ground black pepper
- 1 (1.25-ounce) package dry rib-seasoning rub
- ½ cup sugar-free barbecue sauce

1. With the crock insert in place, preheat the slow cooker to high.
2. Generously season the pork ribs with pink Himalayan salt, pepper, and dry rib-seasoning rub.
3. Stand the ribs up along the walls of the slow-cooker insert, with the bonier side facing inward.
4. Pour the barbecue sauce on both sides of the ribs, using just enough to coat.
5. Cover, cook for 4 hours, and serve.

Kalua Pork With Cabbage

Prep time: 10 minutes|Cook time:8 hours|Serves 2

- Pink Himalayan salt
- Freshly ground black pepper
- 1 tablespoon smoked paprika or Liquid Smoke
- ½ cup water
- ½ head cabbage, chopped

1. With the crock insert in place, preheat the slow cooker to low.
2. Generously season the pork roast with pink Himalayan salt, pepper, and smoked paprika.
3. Place the pork roast in the slow-cooker insert, and add the water.
4. Cover and cook on low for 7 hours.
5. Transfer the cooked pork roast to a plate. Put the chopped cabbage in the bottom of the slow cooker, and put the pork roast back in on top of the cabbage.
6. Cover and cook the cabbage and pork roast for 1 hour.
7. Remove the pork roast from the slow cooker and place it on a baking sheet. Use two forks to shred the pork.
8. Serve the shredded pork hot with the cooked cabbage.
9. Reserve the liquid from the slow cooker to remoisten the pork and cabbage when reheating leftovers.

Blue Cheese Pork Chops

Prep time: 5 minutes|Cook time:10 minutes|Serves 2

- Pink Himalayan salt
- Freshly ground black pepper
- 2 tablespoons butter
- ⅓ cup blue cheese crumbles
- ⅓ cup heavy (whipping) cream
- ⅓ cup sour cream

1. Pat the pork chops dry, and season with pink Himalayan salt and pepper.
2. In a medium skillet over medium heat, melt the butter. When the butter melts and is very hot, add the pork chops and sear on each side for 3 minutes.
3. Transfer the pork chops to a plate and let rest for 3 to 5 minutes.
4. In a medium saucepan over medium heat, melt the blue cheese crumbles, stirring frequently so they don't burn.
5. Add the cream and the sour cream to the pan with the blue cheese. Let simmer for a few minutes, stirring occasionally.
6. For an extra kick of flavor in the sauce, pour the pork-chop pan juice into the cheese mixture and stir. Let simmer while the pork chops are resting.
7. Put the pork chops on two plates, pour the blue cheese sauce over the top of each, and serve.

Pork Burgers With Sriracha Mayo
Prep time: 10 minutes|Cook time:10 minutes|Serves 2

- 2 scallions, white and green parts, thinly sliced
- 1 tablespoon toasted sesame oil
- Pink Himalayan salt
- Freshly ground black pepper
- 1 tablespoon ghee
- 1 tablespoon Sriracha sauce
- 2 tablespoons mayonnaise

1. In a large bowl, mix to combine the ground pork with the scallions and sesame oil, and season with pink Himalayan salt and pepper.
2. Form the pork mixture into 2 patties.
3. Create an imprint with your thumb in the middle of each burger so the pork will heat evenly.
4. In a large skillet over medium-high heat, heat the ghee.
5. When the ghee has melted and is very hot, add the burger patties and cook for 4 minutes on each side.
6. Meanwhile, in a small bowl, mix the Sriracha sauce and mayonnaise.
7. Transfer the burgers to a plate and let rest for at least 5 minutes.
8. Top the burgers with the Sriracha mayonnaise and serve.

Carnitas Nachos
Prep time: 5 minutes|Cook time:10 minutes|Serves 2

- 2 cups pork rinds (I use spicy flavor)
- ½ cup shredded cheese (I use Mexican blend)
- 1 cup Carnitas
- 1 avocado, diced
- 2 tablespoons sour cream

1. Preheat the oven to 350°F. Coat a 9-by-13-inch baking dish with olive oil.
2. Put the pork rinds in the prepared baking dish, and top with the cheese.
3. Put in the oven and bake until the cheese has melted, about 5 minutes. Transfer to a cooling rack and let rest for 5 minutes.
4. In a medium skillet over high heat, heat the olive oil. Put the carnitas in the skillet, and add some of the reserved pan juices. Cook for a few minutes, until you get a nice crispy crust on the carnitas, and then flip the carnitas to the other side and cook briefly.
5. Divide the heated pork rinds and cheese between two plates.
6. Top the pork rinds and cheese with the reheated carnitas, add the diced avocado and a dollop of sour cream to each, and serve hot.

Pepperoni Low-Carb Tortilla Pizza

Prep time: 5 minutes|Cook time:5 minutes|Serves 2

- 2 large low-carb tortillas (I use Mission brand)
- 4 tablespoons low-sugar tomato sauce (I use Rao's)
- 1 cup shredded mozzarella cheese
- 2 teaspoons dried Italian seasoning
- ½ cup pepperoni

1. In a medium skillet over medium-high heat, heat the olive oil.
2. Add the tortilla.
3. Spoon the tomato sauce onto the tortilla, spreading it out.
4. Sprinkle on the cheese, Italian seasoning, and pepperoni.
5. Work quickly so the tortilla doesn't burn.
6. Cook until the tortilla is crispy on the bottom, about 3 minutes.
7. Transfer to a cutting board, and cut into slices.
8. Put the slices on a serving plate and serve hot.

Steak And Egg Bibimbap

Prep time: 10 minutes|Cook time:15 minutes|Serves 2

- 1 tablespoon ghee or butter
- 8 ounces skirt steak
- Pink Himalayan salt
- Freshly ground black pepper
- 1 tablespoon soy sauce (or coconut aminos)
- for the egg and cauliflower rice
- 2 tablespoons ghee or butter, divided
- 2 large eggs
- 1 large cucumber, peeled and cut into matchsticks
- 1 tablespoon soy sauce
- 1 cup cauliflower rice
- Pink Himalayan salt
- Freshly ground black pepper

1. Over high heat, heat a large skillet.
2. Using a paper towel, pat the steak dry.
3. Season both sides with pink Himalayan salt and pepper.
4. Add the ghee or butter to the skillet.
5. When it melts, put the steak in the skillet.
6. Sear the steak for about 3 minutes on each side for medium-rare.
7. Transfer the steak to a cutting board and let it rest for at least 5 minutes.
8. Slice the skirt steak across the grain and divide it between two bowls.
9. to make the egg and cauliflower rice
10. In a second large skillet over medium-high heat, heat 1 tablespoon of ghee.
11. When the ghee is very hot, crack the eggs into it.
12. When the whites have cooked through, after 2 to 3 minutes, carefully transfer the eggs to a plate.
13. In a small bowl, marinate the cucumber matchsticks in the soy sauce.
14. Clean out the skillet from the eggs, and add the remaining 1 tablespoon of ghee or butter to the pan over medium-high heat.
15. Add the cauliflower rice, season with pink Himalayan salt and pepper, and stir, cooking for 5 minutes.
16. Turn the heat up to high at the end of the cooking to get a nice crisp on the "rice."
17. Divide the rice between two bowls.
18. Top the rice in each bowl with an egg, the steak, and the marinated cucumber matchsticks and serve.

Mississippi Pot Roast

Prep time: 5 minutes|Cook time:8 hours|Serves 4

- Pink Himalayan salt
- Freshly ground black pepper
- 1 (1-ounce) packet dry Au Jus Gravy Mix
- 1 (1-ounce) packet dry ranch dressing
- 8 tablespoons butter (1 stick)
- 1 cup whole pepperoncini (I use Mezzetta)

1. With the crock insert in place, preheat the slow cooker to low.
2. Season both sides of the beef chuck roast with pink Himalayan salt and pepper. Put in the slow cooker.
3. Sprinkle the gravy mix and ranch dressing packets on top of the roast.
4. Place the butter on top of the roast, and sprinkle the pepperoncini around it.
5. Cover and cook on low for 8 hours.
6. Shred the beef using two forks, and serve hot.

Taco Cheese Cups

Prep time: 10 minutes|Cook time:20 minutes|Serves 2

- for the cheese cups
- 2 cups shredded cheese (I use Mexican blend)
- for the ground beef
- 1 tablespoon ghee
- ½ pound ground beef
- ½ (1.25-ounce) package taco seasoning
- ¼ cup water
- for the taco cups
- ½ avocado, diced
- Pink Himalayan salt
- Freshly ground black pepper
- 2 tablespoons sour cream

1. Preheat the oven to 350°F.
2. Line a baking sheet with parchment paper or a silicone baking mat.
3. Place ½-cup mounds of the cheese on the prepared pan. Bake for about 7 minutes, or until the edges are brown and the middle has melted.
4. You want these slightly larger than a typical tortilla chip.
5. Put the pan on a cooling rack for 2 minutes while the cheese chips cool.
6. The chips will be floppy when they first come out of the oven, but they will begin to crisp as they cool.
7. Before they are fully crisp, move the cheese chips to a muffin tin.
8. Form the cheese chips around the shape of the muffin cups to create small bowls. (The chips will fully harden in the muffin tin, which will make them really easy to fill.)

TO MAKE THE GROUND BEEF

1. In a medium skillet over medium-high heat, heat the ghee.
2. When the ghee is hot, add the ground beef and sauté for about 8 minutes, until browned.
3. Drain the excess grease.
4. Stir in the taco seasoning and water, and bring to a boil.
5. Turn the heat to medium-low and simmer for 5 minutes.

TO MAKE THE TACO CUPS

1. Using a slotted spoon, spoon the ground beef into the taco cups.
2. Season the diced avocado with pink Himalayan salt and pepper, and divide it among the taco cups.
3. Add a dollop of sour cream to each taco cup and serve.

Lamb Burgers

Prep time: 2 hours|Cook time:15 minutes|Serves 6

- pickled onions
- 1/2 red onion, thinly sliced
- 6 Tbsp [90 ml] lime juice
- 1/2 tsp kosher salt
- 1/2 tsp raw cane sugar
- herbed yogurt sauce
- 1 cup [230 g] Greek yogurt
- 2 Tbsp lemon juice
- 1 garlic clove, minced
- 2 Tbsp finely chopped mixed herbs such as dill, parsley, and mint
- Kosher salt
- lamb burgers
- 1 Tbsp olive oil
- 1/2 red onion, finely diced
- 1 lb [455 g] ground lamb
- 8 oz [230 g] ground pork
- 3 Tbsp finely chopped mint
- 2 Tbsp finely chopped dill
- 3 Tbsp finely chopped parsley
- 4 garlic cloves, minced
- 11/2 tsp ground cumin
- 1 tsp ground coriander
- 1 tsp kosher salt
- 1/2 tsp freshly ground black pepper

1. Mixed greens, sliced tomatoes (optional if nightshade-sensitive), and sliced cucumbers for serving
2. To make the pickled onions: Place the onion, lime juice, salt, and sugar in a small bowl.
3. Stir to combine, cover, and let sit at room temperature for about 2 hours to soften. Refrigerate until ready to use.
4. To make the herbed yogurt sauce: In a small bowl, stir together the yogurt, lemon juice, garlic, herbs, and 1/2 tsp salt.
5. Adjust the salt to taste. Cover and refrigerate until ready to serve, or for up to 2 days.
6. To make the lamb burgers: In a small skillet over medium heat, warm the olive oil.
7. Add the onion and cook, stirring frequently, until softened, about 7 minutes. Transfer to a small plate to cool.
8. In a large bowl, combine the lamb, pork, mint, dill, parsley, garlic, cumin, coriander, salt, pepper, and cooled onions.
9. Gently mix with your hands.
10. Do not overwork the meat. Divide the mixture into six equal balls.
11. Press into patties and transfer to a parchment-lined baking sheet. (If not cooking immediately, cover and refrigerate for up to 8 hours.)
12. Heat a cast-iron skillet over medium-high heat until just smoking.
13. Working in batches, sear the burgers until well browned, 2 to 3 minutes per side for medium-rare, or about 5 minutes per side for well-done.
14. Alternatively, prepare a grill for cooking over medium-high heat. Lightly grease the grill grate.
15. Place the burgers on the grill, and cook, turning once, to reach desired doneness, about 3 minutes per side for medium-rare, or about 5 minutes per side for well-done.
16. Transfer the burgers to a plate to rest for 5 minutes before serving. Top with a generous dollop of herbed yogurt sauce and some pickled onions.
17. Add greens and sliced tomatoes or cucumbers. Serve immediately.
18. how to season burger patties
19. Seasoning meat well is so important.
20. Many times we under- or overseason, then cook the meat and are left with no chance of improving it.
21. Before shaping my patties, I heat a small skillet and cook a test patty, about 1 in [2.5 cm] in diameter, to check for flavor.
22. I adjust the salt and spices if necessary before I form all the patties and cook them.

Carnitas

Prep time: 10 minutes|Cook time:8 hours|Serves 2

- 1 tablespoon olive oil
- 1 pound boneless pork butt roast
- 2 garlic cloves, minced
- ½ small onion, diced
- Pinch pink Himalayan salt
- Pinch freshly ground black pepper
- Juice of 1 lime

1. With the crock insert in place, preheat the slow cooker to low.
2. In a small bowl, mix to combine the chili powder and olive oil, and rub it all over the pork.
3. Place the pork in the slow cooker, fat-side up.
4. Top the pork with the garlic, onion, pink Himalayan salt, pepper, and lime juice.
5. Cover and cook on low for 8 hours.
6. Transfer the pork to a cutting board, shred the meat with two forks, and serve.

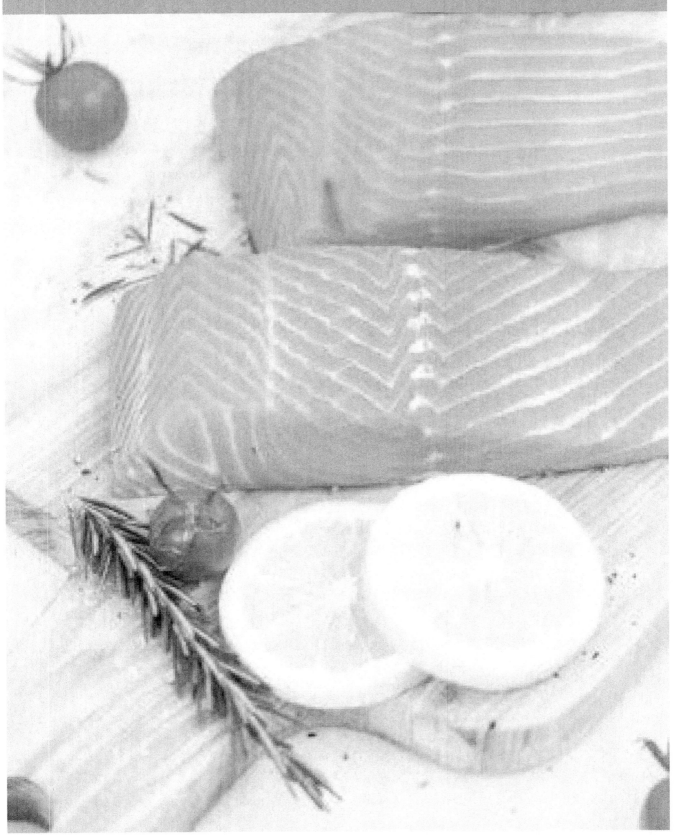

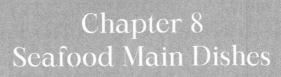

Chapter 8
Seafood Main Dishes

Smoked Haddock & Pea Risotto

Prep time: 4 minutes|Cook time:40 minutes|Serves 2

- 2 smoked haddock fillets skinless, boneless
- 1 tbsp extra virgin olive oil
- 1 white onion, finely diced
- 2 cups brown rice
- 4 cups vegetable stock
- 1 cup fresh spinach leaves
- 1 cup of frozen peas
- 3 tbsp low fat greek yogurt (optional)
- a pinch of black pepper
- 4 lemon wedges
- 1 cup of arugula

1. Heat the oil in a large pan on a medium heat.
2. Sauté the chopped onion for 5 minutes until soft before adding in the rice and stirring for 1-2 minutes.
3. Add half of the stock and stir slowly.
4. Slowly add the rest of the stock whilst continuously stirring for up to 20-30 minutes (this is a bit of a workout!)
5. Stir in the spinach and peas to the risotto.
6. Place the fish on top of the rice, cover and steam for 10 minutes.
7. Use your fork to break up the fish fillets and stir into the rice with the yogurt.
8. Sprinkle with freshly ground pepper to serve and a squeeze of fresh lemon.
9. Garnish with the lemon wedges and serve with the arugula.

Seared Ahi Tuna

Prep time: 15 minutes|Cook time:60 minutes|Serves 4

- One 1-lb [455-g] ahi tuna fillet, about 1 in [2.5 cm] thick
- Extra-virgin olive oil for brushing
- Kosher salt
- Freshly ground black pepper
- 1 cup [210 g] Peperonata

1. Prepare a grill for direct cooking over high heat.
2. Brush the tuna fillet with olive oil and season with salt and pepper.
3. Sear the tuna for 1 to 2 minutes per side for rare, or longer to reach the desired doneness.
4. Transfer to a carving board and let rest for 2 minutes.
5. Slice the tuna against the grain and divide among four plates.
6. Spoon one-fourth of the peperonata over each piece of fish and serve.
7. how to buy tuna
8. My trick to buying good tuna? I always ask the fishmonger to pull a piece from the back for me, not from the display case even if the tuna is right in front of me.
9. The fishmonger should be able to tell you when it came in and should also be happy to cut off a piece from a large, fresh fish.

Shrimp Thermidor

Prep time: 10 minutes|Cook time:12 minutes|Serves 4

- ½ cup ghee or unsalted butter (plus an additional ¼ cup melted ghee or unsalted butter added at the end if using pork rinds)
- 2 cups sliced button mushrooms
- ¼ cup diced onions
- 1 pound large shrimp (about 30), peeled and deveined
- 1 cup chicken bone broth, homemade (here) or store-bought
- 1 (8-ounce) package cream cheese, softened
- ¾ cup shredded cheddar cheese
- 1½ cups crushed pork rinds, divided (optional)
- ½ cup grated Parmesan cheese

1. Preheat the broiler to high.
2. Melt ½ cup of ghee in a cast-iron skillet over medium-high heat.
3. Add the mushrooms and onions and sauté, stirring occasionally, until the mushrooms are golden brown, about 5 minutes.
4. Add the shrimp and sauté for 4 minutes, until the shrimp are cooked through and no longer translucent.
5. Meanwhile, puree the broth and cream cheese in a blender or food processor until smooth, then add the mixture to the skillet.
6. Add the cheddar cheese and stir in 1 cup of the crushed pork rinds, if using.
7. Pour the mixture into a 9-inch square casserole dish.
8. Cover the top of the casserole with the remaining ½ cup of crushed pork rinds, if using, and the Parmesan cheese.
9. If using pork rinds, drizzle ¼ cup of melted ghee over the top.
10. Place under the broiler for 2 to 4 minutes, until the cheese is melted and turning golden brown.
11. Store extras in an airtight container in the refrigerator for up to 4 days.
12. Reheat in a baking dish in a preheated 375°F oven for 4 minutes or until warmed through.

Crispy Fish Tacos

Prep time: 30 minutes|Cook time:10 minutes|Serves 4

- mango salsa
- 2 mangoes, peeled, pitted, and diced
- 1/2 small red onion, finely diced
- 1 jalapeño, minced (optional if nightshade-sensitive)
- 2 Tbsp lime juice, plus more as needed
- 2 Tbsp finely chopped cilantro
- Kosher salt
- avocado crema
- 2 avocados, halved and pitted
- Kosher salt
- 2 Tbsp mayonnaise or Vegenaise
- 2 Tbsp lime juice, plus more as needed

- 1 lb [455 g] tilapia fillets or other white-fleshed fish, such as snapper
- Kosher salt
- Freshly ground black pepper
- 2 eggs
- 1 cup [140 g] Cup4Cup or other gluten-free flour
- 1 cup [30 g] finely grated Parmigiano-Reggiano
- 4 Tbsp [60 ml] extra-virgin olive oil
- 8 corn tortillas, warmed
- 1/2 head red or green cabbage, cored and finely shredded
- Lime wedges for serving

1. To make the mango salsa: Combine the mangos, onion, jalapeño (if using), lime juice, and cilantro in a bowl and stir to combine.
2. Taste, adding salt and lime juice as desired. Set aside.
3. To make the avocado crema: Place the avocado flesh and 1/4 tsp salt in a medium bowl. Using a fork or a pastry blender, mash until very smooth.
4. Stir in the mayonnaise and lime juice.
5. Taste, adding additional salt and lime juice as desired. (Store, with a piece of plastic wrap pressed directly onto the surface, in the refrigerator for up to 2 days.)
6. Rinse the tilapia and pat dry.
7. Halve each fillet lengthwise by slicing down the middle seam. Season with salt and pepper. Whisk the eggs in a shallow bowl.
8. Place the flour, Parmigiano-Reggiano, and 1/2 tsp salt in another small bowl and stir to combine.
9. Dip the fish, one piece at a time, into the eggs, coating evenly and allowing any excess to drip off into the bowl.
10. Then place in the flour mixture and coat both sides evenly, gently tapping off any excess. Arrange the coated fish on a baking sheet in a single layer.
11. Line another baking sheet with paper towels.
12. In a large nonstick skillet over medium-high heat, warm 2 Tbsp of the olive oil.
13. Working in two batches, place the fish pieces in the skillet and cook until golden brown on each side and opaque in the center, about 2 minutes per side.
14. Transfer to the prepared sheet.
15. Pour any remaining oil from the skillet, wipe clean with a paper towel, and add the remaining 2 Tbsp olive oil.
16. Spread some avocado crema on each tortilla.
17. Top with cabbage, a piece of fish, and a spoonful of mango salsa.
18. Serve with lime wedges and extra crema and salsa on the side.

Walleye Simmered in Basil Cream

Prep time: 5 minutes|Cook time:10 minutes|Serves 4

- ¼ cup heavy cream (or full-fat coconut milk if dairy-free)
- ¼ cup fresh basil leaves, plus extra for garnish
- 2 tablespoons ghee or unsalted butter (or coconut oil if dairy-free), divided
- ½ cup chopped onions
- 1 clove garlic, smashed to a paste
- 1 pound walleye fillets, skinned and cut crosswise into 1-inch-wide pieces
- 1 teaspoon fine sea salt
- ¼ teaspoon ground black pepper
- ¼ cup fish or chicken bone broth, homemade or store-bought
- Cherry tomatoes, cut in half, for garnish

1. Place the cream and basil in a food processor or blender and puree until the basil is completely broken down.
2. Heat a cast-iron skillet over medium heat.
3. Melt the ghee in the hot skillet, then add the onions and garlic and sauté for 2 minutes, until the onions are translucent.
4. Season the fish pieces with the salt and pepper.
5. Place the fish in the skillet and add the broth and basil cream. Cook, uncovered, for 7 minutes or until the fish is cooked through and starting to flake.
6. If you prefer a thicker sauce, remove the fish from the pan and continue to boil the sauce for 10 minutes or until thickened to your liking.
7. Place the fish on a serving platter, cover with the sauce, and garnish with additional basil and halved cherry tomatoes.
8. Store extras in an airtight container in the refrigerator for up to 3 days.
9. Reheat in a lightly greased skillet over medium heat until warmed through.

Cheesy Tuna Casserole

Prep time: 10 minutes|Cook time:20 minutes|Serves 6

- 1 tablespoon ghee or unsalted butter (or coconut oil or lard if dairy free), plus extra for greasing the dish
- 1 tablespoon diced celery
- 1 tablespoon diced onions
- 1 clove garlic, smashed to a paste
- 3 (6-ounce) cans tuna, drained
- 2 cups cauliflower florets, cut into ½-inch pieces
- 1 cup chopped dill pickles
- ⅓ cup cream cheese (Kite Hill brand cream cheese style spread if dairy-free), softened
- 2 tablespoons mayonnaise, homemade or store-bought
- ½ teaspoon fine sea salt
- ¼ teaspoon ground black pepper
- 1 cup shredded sharp cheddar cheese (omit for dairy-free)
- Sliced green onions, for garnish
- Chopped fresh parsley, for garnish
- Cherry tomatoes, halved or quartered, depending on size, for garnish

1. Preheat the oven to 375°F. Grease an 11 by 7-inch casserole dish with ghee.
2. Melt 1 tablespoon of ghee in a small skillet over medium-high heat.
3. Add the celery and onions and sauté for 2 to 3 minutes, until the onions are translucent.
4. Add the garlic and sauté for another minute.
5. Move the vegetables to a medium-sized mixing bowl.
6. Add the tuna, cauliflower, pickles, cream cheese, mayonnaise, salt, and pepper to the vegetables and mix to combine.
7. Spoon the tuna mixture into the greased casserole dish.
8. Sprinkle with the cheddar cheese, if using. Bake for 20 minutes or until the cauliflower is tender and the casserole is lightly browned on top.
9. Remove from the oven and allow to stand for 5 minutes. Serve garnished with green onions, parsley, and cherry tomatoes.
10. This dish is best served fresh, but any leftovers can be stored in an airtight container in the refrigerator for up to 3 days.
11. Reheat in a baking dish in a preheated 350°F oven for 3 minutes or until warmed through.

Smoked Salmon Hash Browns

Prep time: 5 minutes|Cook time:35 minutes|Serves 4

- 1 large sweet potato, peeled and cubed
- 3 tbsp extra virgin olive oil
- 1 leek, chopped
- 4 tsp dill, chopped
- 1 tbsp grated orange peel
- 1 pack smoked salmon, sliced
- 1`/3 cup low fat greek yogurt
- (optional)

1. Preheat oven to 325°F/150°C/Gas Mark 3.
2. Lightly grease 2 ramekins or circular baking dishes with a little olive oil.
3. Heat the rest of the oil in a skillet over medium heat, and sauté the leeks and the potatoes for 5 minutes.
4. Lower the heat and cook for another 10 minutes until tender.
5. Transfer the potatoes and leeks to a separate bowl and crush with a fork to form a mash (alternatively use a potato masher).
6. Add the dill, orange peel and the salmon and mix well.
7. Fill the ramekins with half the mixture each, patting to compact.
8. Bake for 15 minutes and remove.
9. Serve in the ramekin, season and top with a dollop of Greek yogurt (optional).

Charleston Shrimp 'n' Gravy Over Grits

Prep time: 5 minutes|Cook time:15 minutes|Serves 4

- 3 strips bacon
- 2 tablespoons ghee or unsalted butter
- 1 green bell pepper, chopped
- ½ cup diced onions
- 1 clove garlic, smashed to a paste or minced
- 1 pound large shrimp (about 30), peeled and deveined
- 2 teaspoons fine sea salt
- ½ teaspoon ground black pepper
- ½ cup chicken bone broth, homemade or store-bought
- Double batch Keto Grits, for serving

1. Fry the bacon in a cast-iron skillet over medium-high heat until crisp, about 4 minutes.
2. Remove from the skillet and set aside. Leave the drippings in the pan.
3. Add the ghee to the skillet with the bacon drippings and reduce the heat to medium.
4. Add the bell pepper and onions and sauté for 5 minutes or until the onions are soft.
5. Add the garlic and cook for another minute.
6. Season the shrimp with the salt and pepper.
7. Add the shrimp to the skillet, increase the heat to medium-high, and sauté, stirring constantly, for about 4 minutes, until the shrimp are no longer translucent.
8. Using a slotted spoon, remove the shrimp to a warm plate and set aside.
9. Add the broth to the skillet, still over medium-high heat, and whisk the bottom of the skillet to deglaze.
10. Boil the broth until it is thickened to your liking, then remove the skillet from the heat, add the shrimp to the sauce, and stir to coat.
11. Serve the shrimp over keto grits, with the bacon crumbled on top.
12. Store extras in an airtight container in the refrigerator for up to 3 days.
13. Reheat in a lightly greased skillet over medium heat until warmed through.

Seafood Risotto

Prep time: 10 minutes|Cook time:7 minutes|Serves 4

- 1 medium head cauliflower, cored and separated into florets
- 2 tablespoons ghee, unsalted butter, or coconut oil
- 2 tablespoons diced onions
- 1 clove garlic, finely chopped
- 4 ounces mascarpone or cream cheese (½ cup)
- Fine sea salt and ground black pepper
- ½ cup chicken bone broth, homemade (here) or store-bought
- ¼ cup grated Parmesan cheese
- 2 cups cooked whole shrimp or cooked crab or langostino pieces

1. To make the "rice," place the cauliflower florets in a food processor and pulse until the cauliflower is rice-sized; set aside.
2. Heat the ghee in a cast-iron skillet over medium heat.
3. When hot, add the onions and garlic and sauté for 2 minutes, stirring often.
4. Add the cauliflower rice and mascarpone and season with a couple of pinches each of salt and pepper.
5. Whisk and cook the mixture until the mascarpone is soft, about 1 minute.
6. Add the broth slowly, while whisking. Cook for 4 minutes or until the "rice" is soft.
7. Add the Parmesan cheese and cooked shrimp and stir to combine; cook for a minute or two to heat through, then season to taste with salt and pepper, if needed, and serve.
8. Store extras in an airtight container in the refrigerator for up to 3 days.
9. Reheat in a lightly greased skillet over medium heat until warmed through.

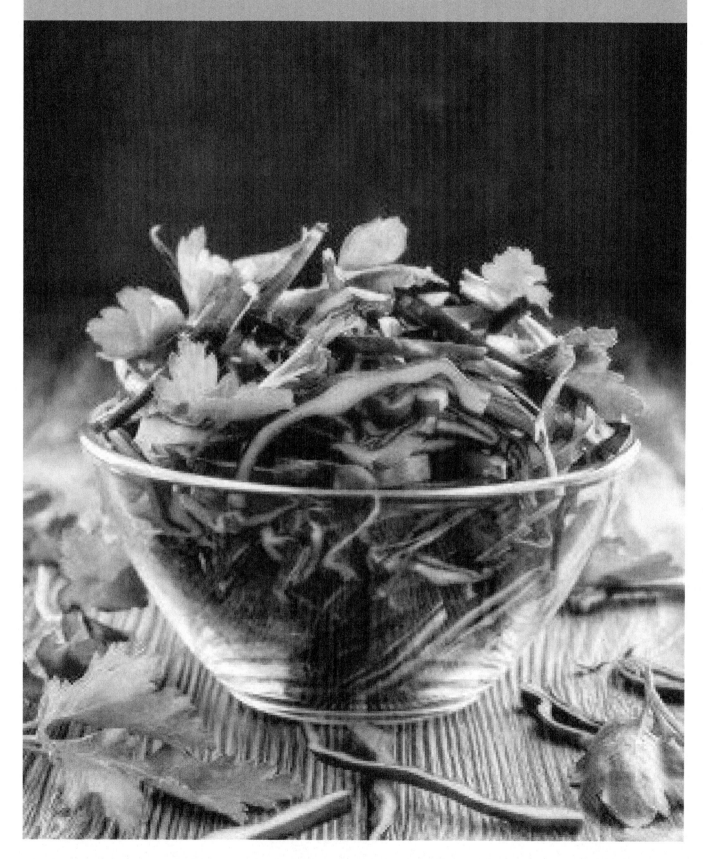

Chapter 9
Salads And Sides

Roasted Beetroot, Goats' Cheese & Egg Salad

Prep time: 2 minutes|Cook time:25 minutes|Serves 1

- 1/2 cup cooked chopped beetroot (not in vinegar)
- 2 tbsp extra virgin olive oil
- juice from 1 orange
- 1 free range egg
- 2 tbsp low fat greek yogurt
- 1 tsp dijon mustard
- a few stalks of dill, finely chopped (fresh or dried)
- 1/2 cup of baby gem lettuce
- handful of walnuts
- 1/4 cup crumbled goats cheese
- a pinch black pepper

1. Preheat oven to 200°C/400°F/Gas Mark 6.
2. Place the beetroot onto a lightly oiled baking tray with the juice from the orange and sprinkle with pepper.
3. Roast for 20-25 minutes, turning once whilst baking. If it starts to dry out, add a little more olive oil.
4. Meanwhile, boil a pan of water and add the whole egg.
5. Turn down the heat and simmer for 8 minutes (4 minutes if you like your yolks runny) then run under cold water to cool. Peel and halve.
6. Mix the remaining oil, yogurt, mustard and chopped dill together - this is the dressing for your lettuce.
7. Serve the salad with the beetroot and goats' cheese and walnuts crumbled over the top.

Kipper & Celery Salad

Prep time: 2 minutes|Cook time:0 minutes|Serves 2

- 1 can of cooked kippers
- 1 celery stalk, chopped
- 1 tbsp fresh parsley, chopped
- 1/2 cup low fat greek yogurt
- 1 lemon, juiced
- 1 clove garlic, minced
- 1 onion, minced

1. Combine all of the ingredients apart from the kippers into a salad bowl.
2. Drain the kippers and then toss in the dressing mix.
3. Chill before serving for at least 20 minutes in the fridge.
4. Top tip: If you have mackerel or sardines, this works just as well.

Cumin & Mango Chicken Salad

Prep time: 30 minutes|Cook time:15 minutes|Serves 2

- 2 free range skinless chicken breasts
- 1 tsp oregano, finely chopped
- 1 garlic clove, minced
- 1 tsp chili flakes
- 1 tsp cumin
- 1 tsp turmeric
- 1 tbsp extra virgin olive oil
- 1 lime, juiced
- 1 cup mango, cubed
- 1/2 iceberg/romaine lettuce or
- similar, sliced

1. In a bowl mix oil, garlic, herbs and spices with the lime juice.
2. Add the chicken and marinate for at least 30 minutes up to overnight.
3. When ready to serve, preheat the broiler to a medium high heat.
4. Add the chicken to a lightly greased baking tray and broil for 10-12 minutes or until cooked through.
5. Combine the lettuce with the mango in a serving bowl.
6. Once the chicken is cooked, serve immediately on top of the mango and lettuce.

Japanese Avocado & Shrimp Salad

Prep time: 2 minutes|Cook time:4 minutes|Serves 2

- 1 garlic clove, minced
- 2 cups of raw shrimp, with the
- tails removed
- 1/2 tbsp extra virgin olive oil
- 1/2 tsp chili powder
- 1/4 tsp cayenne
- 1 avocado, sliced
- 1/2 cucumber, chopped
- 2 cups spinach or baby kale,
- washed and chopped
- for the miso dressing:
- 1 thumb sized piece of fresh ginger, finely chopped
- 2 tbsp extra virgin olive oil
- 3 tbsp lime juice
- 2 tbsp agave nectar/honey
- 1 tbsp white miso (available from most grocery stores)
- 1/2 tsp minced garlic

1. Heat the oil in a skillet over a medium heat, adding in the garlic and shrimp, and then sprinkle with chili powder and cayenne.
2. Sauté for 8-10 minutes or until shrimp cooked through.
3. Cut the avocadoes in half and scoop out the flesh.
4. Dice the cucumber, and chop the baby spinach and kale into small spices.
5. Arrange in a bowl with the cooked shrimp.
6. Put all of the ingredients for the dressing into a food processor and process until smooth.
7. Pour over the salad and serve immediately, topping with cilantro and peanuts for an extra crunch!

Mustard Cauliflower Slices

Prep time: 5 minutes|Cook time:0 minutes|Serves 2

- 2 cups cauliflower florets, finely sliced
- for the dressing:
- 1 tsp extra virgin olive oil
- 1 lemon, juiced
- 1 large garlic clove, minced
- 1 tsp wholegrain mustard

1. Get a large salad bowl and combine all of the ingredients.
2. Serve immediately so that the cauliflower remains crunchy!

Egg & Mixed Bean Salad

Prep time: 30 minutes|Cook time:0 minutes|Serves 4

- 1/2½cup of cooked black beans
- 1/2 cup of cooked cannellini beans
- 1/2 cup of cooked kidney beans
- 2 hard-boiled eggs, sliced
- 1 celery stick, chopped
- 2 green onions, chopped
- 8 green olives, pitted and sliced
- 1/2 tsp of black pepper
- 3 tsp extra virgin olive oil
- 1 tsp dried oregano

1. Rinse and drain the beans.
2. Combine celery, olives, olive oil, herbs and beans in a serving bowl and mix.
3. Refrigerate for at least 30 minutes.
4. When ready to serve, add the halved boiled eggs.
5. Sprinkle over chopped green onions and enjoy.

Cashew Nuts & Broccoli Snack

Prep time: 5 minutes|Cook time:25 minutes|Serves 4

- 1/2 cup cashews
- 1/2¼ cup water
- 2 tbsp yellow curry powder
- pinch of pepper
- 4 cups broccoli, sliced
- 2 tbsp sunflower seeds

1. Preheat oven to the highest heat.
2. Layer the cashew nuts onto a dry baking tray and add to the oven for 5-10 minutes or until nuts start to brown. Turn whilst cooking to ensure even browning.
3. Remove to cool.
4. Meanwhile boil a pan of water on a medium heat and add the broccoli.
5. Cook on a simmer for 5-10 minutes or until cooked through.
6. Drain and place to one side.
7. Blend the water, curry powder, pepper and sunflower seeds until smooth.
8. Crush the cashew nuts on a wooden chopping board or similar, using a sharp knife.
9. When ready to serve, dress the broccoli with the sesame dressing, and top with roasted cashew nuts.

Baked Apple & Walnut Chips

Prep time: 5 minutes|Cook time:30 minutes|Serves 4

- 4 apples, peeled and thinly sliced
- 1 tbsp cinnamon
- 1/4 cup of walnut pieces for topping

1. Preheat oven to 190°C/375°F/Gas Mark 5.
2. Layer the apple slices in a thin layer on a baking tray.
3. Dust with the cinnamon and top with walnut pieces.
4. Bake for 20-30 minutes or until crispy.

Homemade Moroccan Hummus

Prep time: 5 minutes|Cook time:0 minutes|Serves 4

- for the hummus:
- 1 can of chickpeas
- 2 cloves of garlic, minced
- 1 tbsp tahini paste
- 4 tbsp extra virgin olive oil
- 1 tsp ground cumin
- 1 tsp turmeric
- 1 tsp harissa
- 1 tsp salt
- 1 lemon, juiced
- to serve:
- 1/8 red onion, finely chopped
- 1/2 beef tomato, finely chopped
- 1 tsp extra virgin olive oil

1. Take all of the ingredients for the hummus and add to a food processor, processing until smooth (leave a little chunky for a rustic finish or add a little water to loosen the consistency if required).
2. Transfer to a serving dish and create a shallow well in the middle with your spoon.
3. Top with the red onion and tomato combined and drizzle with the remaining oil to serve.
4. Sprinkle with a little black pepper to taste and serve as a dip for your favorite veggies or even as a side with your couscous, quinoa or favorite fish or meat dish.

Brilliantly Beetroot Flavoured Ketchup

Prep time: 5 minutes|Cook time:45 minutes|Serves 2

- 2 whole beetroots
- 1 juiced lemon
- 4 tbsp sunflower seeds, soaked overnight
- 1 tsp mustard powder
- a pinch of black pepper to taste

1. Preheat oven 350°F/180 °C/Gas Mark 4.
2. Bake the beetroot for 30-40 minutes or until tender, and then peel and chop into cubes.
3. Add the rest of the ingredients and the beetroot into a blender and puree until smooth.

Zainy Zucchini Ketchup

Prep time: 15 minutes|Cook time:0 minutes|Serves 4

- 2 zucchinis, peeled and sliced
- 1/2½cup fresh parsley
- 2 tbsp lemon juice
- 1 tbsp extra virgin olive oil
- 1 garlic clove, minced
- a pinch of black pepper
- 2 tbsp chopped walnuts

1. Allow zucchini to dry out a little by slicing and placing on kitchen towel to soak up the moisture for 10 minutes or longer if possible.
2. Process the zucchini with the rest of the ingredients (apart from the nuts) until smooth.
3. Fold in the nuts to the mixture and then refrigerate for at least 10 minutes before serving with your favorite crudites or sweet potato fries.

Rustic Apricot & Walnut Rice

Prep time: 5 minutes|Cook time:25 minutes|Serves 2

- 1/2 cup walnuts
- 2 cups homemade chicken broth
- 1 cup uncooked brown rice
- 1 tbsp extra virgin olive oil
- 1 onion, chopped
- 1/1 cup dried apricots
- 1 orange, zest and juice

1. Preheat oven to 375°F/190 °C/Gas Mark 5.
2. Layer walnuts on a baking tray and roast for 10 minutes.
3. Meanwhile, put the broth and brown rice into a saucepan and boil on a high heat.
4. Reduce the heat and simmer for 25 minutes until rice is cooked and the broth is absorbed.
5. Meanwhile, heat the oil in a skillet on a medium heat and sauté the onion until soft.
6. Add the apricots and cook for another 10 minutes.
7. Stir in the walnuts and the orange zest and juice, and then fold the mixture into the rice, adding pepper to taste.

Mustard & Tarragon Sweet Potato Salad

Prep time: 5 minutes|Cook time:30 minutes|Serves 2

- 2 medium sized sweet potatoes, peeled and cubed
- 1/2½cup of low-fat greek yogurt
- 2 tbsp of dijon mustard
- 1 tbsp dried tarragon
- 1 beef tomato, finely chopped
- (retain the seeds) – optional
- 1/2½yellow pepper, finely chopped
- – optional
- 1/2 red onion, finely chopped
- pinch of black pepper to taste

1. Boil water in a large pot on a high heat.
2. Cook the potatoes in the pot for 20 minutes or until tender.
3. Set aside after draining to cool down.
4. Combine Dijon mustard, plain yogurt, tarragon, peppers, tomatoes and red onion in a serving bowl.
5. Add the cooled potatoes and mix well.
6. Enjoy!

Roasted Paprika Pumpkin Seeds

Prep time: 5 minutes|Cook time:15 minutes|Serves 4

- 1 cup pumpkin seeds
- 1 tbsp extra virgin olive oil
- 1 tsp paprika
- 1 tsp chili powder
- 1 tsp dried oregano

1. Preheat oven to 375°F/190 °C/Gas Mark 5.
2. Layer the seeds on a baking tray.
3. Combine the oil, paprika, oregano and the chili powder together and coat the pumpkin seeds evenly.
4. Bake for 15 minutes and serve.

Sweet And Salty Nuts

Prep time: 2 minutes|Cook time:20 minutes|Serves 4

- 2 cups of unsalted mixed nuts – pecans, peanuts and almonds
- 1 free range egg white
- 1 tbsp honey
- 1 tsp coconut oil for cooking
- 1 tsp black pepper
- 1 pinch chili powder

1. Preheat oven to 375°F/190 °C/Gas Mark 5.
2. In a pan add the egg white, chili, pepper and honey and heat on a low heat for 3 minutes.
3. Put the nuts into the pan and then coat them with the mixture.
4. Once ready, spread the nuts into a single layer on a baking sheet and then bake for at least 15 minutes.
5. Be careful they don't burn by turning half way through.
6. Remove and cool before serving.

Spiced Apple & Quince Sauce

Prep time: 5 minutes|Cook time:40 minutes|Serves 2

- 2 quinces, peeled, cored and diced
- 4 cups cooking apples, cut into chunks
- 1 orange, juiced
- 1 cinnamon stick

1. Put the quinces and apples in a large pan of water on a medium heat and simmer for 30-40 minutes or until tender (your fork should go right through and crumble the apple).
2. Add to the blender with the rest of the ingredients and whizz up until pureed.
3. You can serve hot or cold with your favorite snacks.

Salade Niçoise

Prep time: 30 minutes|Cook time:40 minutes|Serves 2

- 2 baby beets, peeled and cut into large dice
- 2 Tbsp extra-virgin olive oil
- 8 oz [230 g] green beans, trimmed
- Four 4-oz [115-g] skin-on salmon fillets, pin bones removed
- Kosher salt
- French Vinaigrette
- Freshly ground black pepper
- 1 cup [180 g] halved cherry tomatoes (optional if nightshade-sensitive)
- 3 hard-boiled eggs, quartered
- 1/2 cup [70 g] oil-cured Niçoise olives, pitted
- 1 Tbsp minced chives

1. Preheat the oven to 400°F [200°C].
2. In a small roasting pan, toss the beets with 1 Tbsp of the olive oil. Roast, stirring every 10 to 15 minutes, until the beets are soft and caramelized, about 40 minutes. Set aside to cool.
3. Bring a pot of salted water to a boil and fill a medium bowl with ice water.
4. Add the green beans to the boiling water and cook for 2 minutes.
5. With a slotted spoon, transfer the beans to the ice-water bath to stop the cooking.
6. Be careful not to overcook the beans, they should still have some bite. Dry the beans.
7. Rinse the salmon and pat dry with a paper towel.
8. Sprinkle each side with a small pinch of salt.
9. Place a medium nonstick sauté pan over medium-high heat.
10. When the pan is hot, add the remaining 1 Tbsp olive oil. Place the salmon fillets skin-side down in the pan and cook until the skin is crispy, about 2 minutes.
11. For medium-rare salmon, turn the fillets and cook for 1 minute more.
12. For medium salmon, also turn the salmon on its sides, cooking each side for 1 minute.
13. Remove and place on a wire rack so the skin doesn't get soggy.
14. Place the green beans in a medium bowl, add 1 Tbsp of the vinaigrette, and toss to coat.
15. Taste and add a pinch of salt and pepper if needed.
16. Arrange the beans in a pile on a serving platter.
17. Repeat with the beets and cherry tomatoes (if using).
18. Add the hard-boiled eggs and olives to the platter, then top with the salmon fillets.
19. Drizzle with a little vinaigrette, then sprinkle with the chives. Serve family style.

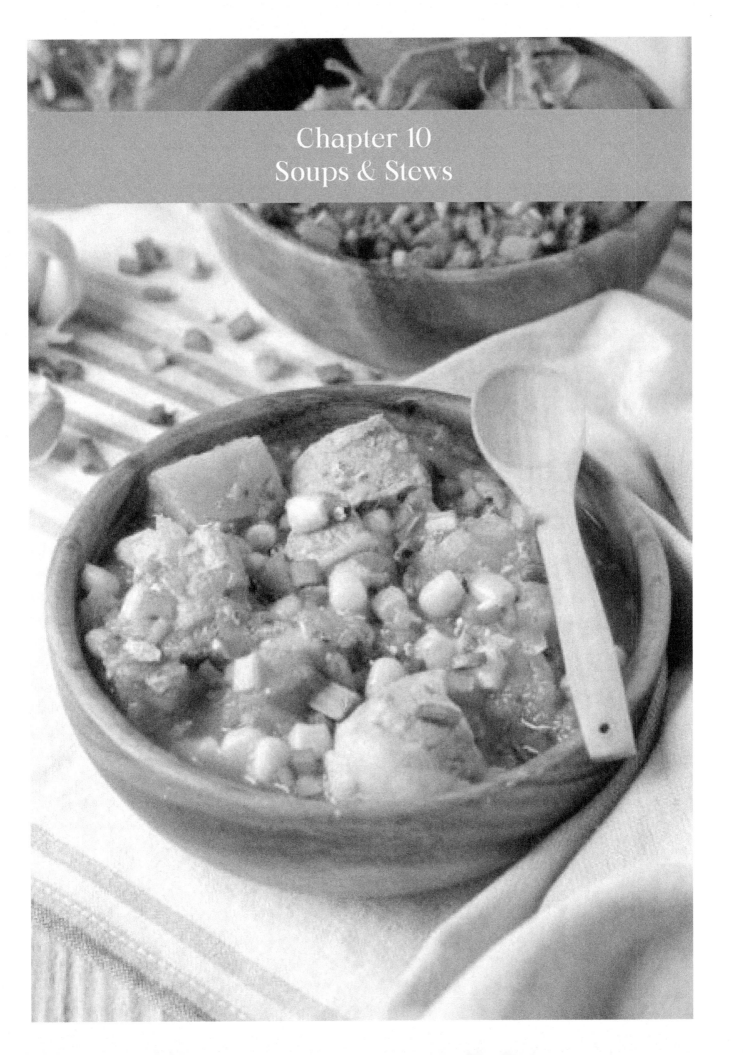

Chapter 10
Soups & Stews

Ginger, Carrot & Lime Soup

Prep time: 5 minutes|Cook time:40 minutes|Serves 2

- 2 tbsp olive oil
- 1 tsp mustard seeds, ground
- 1 tsp coriander seeds, ground
- 1 tsp curry powder
- 1 tbsp ginger, minced
- 4 cups carrots, thinly sliced
- 2 cups onions, chopped
- zest and juice of 1 lime
- 4 cups low-salt vegetable broth
- black pepper for taste

1. In a pan on a medium heat, heat the oil, and add the seeds and curry powder for 1 minute.
2. Add the ginger and then cook for another minute.
3. Then add in the carrots, onions, and the lime zest, cooking for at least 2 minutes or until the vegetables are soft.
4. Add the broth and allow to boil before turning heat down slightly and allowing to simmer for 30 minutes.
5. Allow to cool.
6. Put the mixture in a food processor and puree until smooth.
7. Serve with lime juice and black pepper.

Asian Squash & Shitake Soup

Prep time: 10 minutes|Cook time:45 minutes|Serves 2

- 15 dried shiitake mushrooms, soaked in water
- 6 cups low salt vegetable stock
- 1/2 butternut squash, peeled and cubed
- 1 tbsp sesame oil
- 1 onion, quartered and sliced into rings
- 1 large garlic clove, chopped
- 4 stems of pak choy or equivalent
- 1 sprig of thyme or 1 tbsp. dried thyme
- 1 tsp tabasco sauce (optional)

1. Heat sesame oil in a large pan on a medium high heat before sweating the onions and garlic.
2. Add the vegetable stock and bring to a boil over a high heat before adding the squash.
3. Turn down heat and allow to simmer for 25-30 minutes.
4. Soak the mushrooms in the water if not already done, and then press out the liquid and add to the stock into the pot.
5. Use the mushroom water in the stock for extra taste.
6. Add the rest of the ingredients except for the greens and allow to simmer for a further 15 minutes or until the squash is tender.
7. Add in the chopped greens and let them wilt before serving. Serve with the tabasco sauce if you like it spicy.

Tasty Thai Broth

Prep time: 5 minutes|Cook time:25 minutes|Serves 2

- 2 tbsp olive oil
- 1 tbsp sesame oil
- 1 tbsp cilantro seeds
- 1 red chili, finely chopped
- a handful of fresh basil leaves
- 2 skinless cod pieces
- 2 fresh limes
- 1 garlic clove
- 1 thumb size piece of minced ginger
- 1 white onion, chopped
- 2 handfuls baby spinach leaves
- 1 pac choi (leaves pulled off)
- separately but not sliced)
- 1/2 cup of homemade chicken broth
- 1/2 cup of coconut milk
- 1 red chili, finely chopped

1. Crush the cilantro seeds, chili and basil in a blender or pestle and mortar.
2. Mix in 1 tbsp of olive oil until a paste is formed.
3. Heat a large pan/wok with sesame oil on a high heat.
4. Fry the onions, garlic and ginger for 5-6 minutes until soft but not crispy or browned.
5. Add the spice paste with the coconut milk into the pan and stir.
6. Slowly add the stock until a broth is formed.
7. Now add your fish pieces and allow to simmer in the broth for 10-15 minutes or until cooked through.
8. Add the pak choi, basil and spinach 2-3 minutes before the end of the cooking time.
9. Serve with the fresh lime wedges.

Beef Stew

Prep time: 15 minutes|Cook time:1 hour 40 minutes|Serves 8

- 1 (1-pound) boneless beef roast
- Fine sea salt and ground black pepper
- 3 tablespoons MCT oil or bacon fat
- ½ head (2 cups) cauliflower, cut into 1-inch pieces
- 2 cups button mushrooms, sliced in half
- 1 cup diced onions
- 2 large stalks celery, cut into ¼-inch pieces
- 3 cloves garlic, minced, or 1 head roasted garlic, cloves squeezed from the head
- 4 cups beef bone broth, homemade (here) or store-bought
- 1 (28-ounce) can diced tomatoes, or 2 fresh tomatoes, diced
- ½ teaspoon dried rosemary, or 1 teaspoon fresh rosemary, finely chopped
- ½ teaspoon dried thyme, or 1 teaspoon fresh thyme, finely chopped

1. Pat the roast dry with a paper towel and cut it into 1-inch pieces. Season the meat on all sides with salt and pepper.
2. Place the MCT oil in a Dutch oven over medium-high heat.
3. When hot, sear the beef chunks in the oil until they are golden brown on all sides, about 3 minutes.
4. Add the cauliflower, mushrooms, onions, celery, and garlic to the pot with the beef. Sauté for 3 minutes.
5. Add the broth, tomatoes, rosemary, and thyme to the pot.
6. Cover and cook for 1 hour, stirring every 20 minutes or so.
7. Uncover and cook for another 30 minutes to thicken the stew. Remove from the heat and serve.
8. Store extras in an airtight container in the refrigerator for up to 4 days or in the freezer for up to 1 month.
9. Reheat in a saucepan over medium heat for 5 minutes or until warmed through.

Moroccan Spiced Lentil Soup

Prep time: 5 minutes|Cook time:40 minutes|Serves 2

- 2 tbsp extra virgin olive oil
- 1 yellow onion, diced
- 1 carrots, diced
- 1 cloves of minced garlic, diced
- 1 tsp ground cumin
- 1/2 tsp ground ginger
- 2 tbsp low fat greek yogurt
- 1/2 tsp ground turmeric
- 1/2 tsp red chili flakes
- 1 can chopped tomatoes
- 1 cup dried yellow lentils, soaked
- 5 cups of low salt vegetable stock or homemade chicken stock
- 1 lemon

1. In a large pan, heat the oil on a medium high heat.
2. Sauté the onion and carrot for 5-6 minutes , until softened and starting to brown.
3. Add the garlic, ginger, chili flakes, cumin and turmeric, cooking for 2 minutes.
4. Add the tomatoes, scraping any brown bits from the bottom of the pan and cooking until the liquid is reduced (15-20 minutes).
5. Add the lentils and stock and turn the heat up to reach a boil before lowering heat, covering and then simmering for 10 minutes.
6. Serve with a wedge of lemon on the side and a dollop of Greek yogurt.

Winter Warming Chunky Chicken Soup

Prep time: 7 minutes|Cook time:40 minutes|Serves 7

- 1 whole free range chicken (no giblets), cooked
- 1 bay leaf
- 5 cups of homemade chicken broth/water
- 1 onion, chopped
- 2 stalks of celery, sliced
- 3 carrots, chopped and peeled
- 2 parsnips, chopped and peeled
- sprinkle of pepper to season

1. Add all of the ingredients minus the pepper into a large pot and boil on a high heat.
2. Once boiling, lower the heat and allow to simmer for 30 minutes, or until the chicken is piping hot throughout.
3. Remove the chicken and place on a chopping board.
4. Slice as much meat as you can from the chicken and remove the skin and bones.
5. Add it back into the pot and either serve right away as a chunky soup or allow to cool and whizz through the blender to serve.
6. Add black pepper to season and serve alone or with your choice of wholegrain bread – quinoa tastes delicious with this too – just pop it into the soup 20 minutes before the end and it will soak up all the delicious flavors.

Cream of Chicken Soup

Prep time: 10 minutes|Cook time:35 minutes|Serves 4

- 2 cups chicken bone broth, home made (here) or store-bought
- ½ cup diced celery
- 4 ounces cream cheese (½ cup) (Kite Hill brand cream cheese style spread if dairy-free), softened
- 1 tablespoon ghee or unsalted butter (or coconut oil or bacon fat if dairy-free)
- 2 tablespoons minced shallots
- 2 cloves garlic, smashed to a paste
- 2 boneless, skinless chicken thighs, chopped into ¼-inch pieces
- 1 teaspoon dried thyme leaves
- 1 teaspoon fine sea salt
- ½ teaspoon ground black pepper
- ½ bay leaf
- 1 tablespoon lemon juice, or more to taste
- Fresh herbs of choice, such as oregano or thyme, for garnish
- Avocado oil or extra-virgin olive oil, for drizzling

1. In a food processor, puree the broth, celery, and softened cream cheese. Set aside.
2. Melt the ghee in a saucepan over medium heat.
3. Add the shallots and garlic and lightly sauté for 2 minutes, until fragrant.
4. Add the chopped chicken and sauté for 6 minutes or until the chicken is cooked through and no longer pink.
5. Add the celery puree, thyme, salt, pepper, and bay leaf to the soup and cook over medium heat for 25 minutes.
6. Remove the bay leaf. Stir in the lemon juice.
7. Taste and add more salt, pepper, or lemon juice, if desired. Serve garnished with fresh herbs and a drizzle of oil.
8. Store extras in an airtight container in the refrigerator for up to 3 days.
9. Reheat in a saucepan over medium heat for a few minutes or until warmed through.

Mushroom Truffle Bisque

Prep time: 5 minutes|Cook time:10 minutes|Serves 4

- 2 tablespoons unsalted butter or ghee (or coconut oil if dairy-free)
- 4 ounces button mushrooms, sliced
- 4 ounces baby portobello mushrooms, sliced
- ¼ cup chopped white onions
- ½ teaspoon fine sea salt
- 1 clove garlic, minced
- 2 cups chicken bone broth, homemade (here) or store-bought
- 1 (8-ounce) package cream cheese (Kite Hill brand cream cheese style spread if dairy-free), softened
- Diced cooked bacon, for garnish (optional)
- 1 teaspoon truffle oil, for drizzling (optional)

1. Melt the butter in a stockpot or large saucepan over medium heat.
2. Add the mushrooms and onions and sauté until the onions are translucent, about 4 minutes. Season with the salt.
3. Add the garlic and sauté for another minute.
4. Remove some of the mushrooms and reserve for garnish.
5. Add the broth and cream cheese to the pot and heat through.
6. Use an immersion blender to puree the soup. Ladle into serving bowls and garnish each bowl with a few of the reserved mushrooms, some diced cooked bacon, and a drizzle of truffle oil, if desired.
7. Store extras in an airtight container in the refrigerator for up to 3 days.
8. Reheat in a saucepan over medium heat for a few minutes or until warmed through.

Fauxtato Leek Soup

Prep time: 5 minutes|Cook time:25 minutes|Serves 6

- 4 strips bacon, diced
- ½ cup chopped leeks
- ½ cup diced celery
- 2 cups cauliflower florets and chunked cauliflower stem, about ½ inch in size
- 2 cups chicken bone broth, homemade or store-bought
- 1 (8-ounce) package cream cheese (Kite Hill brand cream cheese style spread if dairy-free), softened
- ½ teaspoon fish sauce (optional)
- 1½ teaspoons fine sea salt
- ½ teaspoon ground black pepper
- Avocado oil or extra-virgin olive oil, for drizzling
- Fresh thyme leaves, for garnish

1. In a large saucepan or Dutch oven, fry the bacon over medium-high heat until crisp, about 4 minutes.
2. Remove the bacon and set aside, leaving the drippings in the pan.
3. Add the leeks, celery, and cauliflower pieces to the pan. Sauté for 5 minutes or until the leeks are soft.
4. Pour in the chicken broth and cook over medium heat until the veggies are tender, about 10 minutes.
5. Place ½ cup of the cooked cauliflower mixture and the cream cheese in a food processor and puree until smooth. (This will help thicken the soup.)
6. Return the puree to the pan with the vegetables. Stir in the fish sauce (if using), salt, and pepper.
7. Taste and adjust the seasoning as desired. Heat through, but do not allow the soup to boil.
8. Serve the soup drizzled with oil and garnished with thyme and the reserved bacon.
9. Store extras in an airtight container in the refrigerator for up to 3 days.
10. Reheat in a saucepan over medium heat for a few minutes or until warmed through.

Spiced Red Pepper & Tomato Soup

Prep time: 2 minutes|Cook time:35 minutes|Serves 2

- 2 red bell peppers
- 4 beef tomatoes
- 1 sweet onion, chopped
- 1 garlic clove, chopped
- 3 cups homemade chicken broth
- 2 habanero chilis with the stems removed and chopped
- 2 tbsp of extra virgin olive oil

1. Preheat the broiler to a medium high heat and grill the bell peppers, turning half way until the skins are blackened for 10 minutes.
2. Meanwhile, heat water in a pan on a medium to high heat and cut a small x at the bottom of each tomato using a sharp knife.
3. Transfer peppers once cooked to a separate dish and cover.
4. Blanch the tomatoes in simmering water for about 20 seconds.
5. Remove and plunge into ice cold water.
6. Peel and chop tomatoes, reserving the juices.
7. Saute the onion, garlic, chils and 2 tbsp of oil in a saucepan on a medium high heat, stirring until golden for 8-10 minutes.
8. Add the tomatoes with the juices, the peppers and broth to the onions and cover and simmer for 10-15 minutes or until heated through.
9. Puree in a blender and serve.

Flavorsome Vegetarian Tagine

Prep time: 10 minutes|Cook time:45 minutes|Serves 2

- 2 tbsp coconut oil
- 1 onion, diced
- 1 parsnip, peeled and diced
- 2 cloves of garlic
- 1 tsp ground cumin
- 1/2 tsp ground ginger
- 1/2 tsp ground cinnamon
- 1/4 tsp cayenne pepper
- 3 tbsp tomato paste
- 1 sweet potato, peeled & diced
- 1 purple potato, peeled & diced
- 4 baby carrots, peeled & diced
- 4 cups low-salt vegetable stock
- 2 cups kale leaves
- 2 tbsp lemon juice
- 1/4 cup cilantro, roughly chopped
- handful of toasted almonds

1. In a large pot, heat the oil on a medium high heat before sautéing the onion until soft.
2. Add the parsnip for 10 minutes or until golden brown.
3. Add the garlic, cumin, ginger, cinnamon, tomato paste, and cayenne.
4. Cook for about 2 minutes until the lovely scents reach your nose.
5. Fold in the sweet potatoes, carrots, and the purple potatoes and stock and then bring to a boil.
6. Turn heat down and simmer for 20 minutes.
7. Add in the kale and lemon juice, simmering for a further 2 minutes or until the leaves are slightly wilted.
8. Garnish with the cilantro and the nuts to serve.

Chicken "Wild Rice" Soup

Prep time: 20 minutes|Cook time:1/2 hours|Serves 10

- ½ cup (1 stick) unsalted butter (or lard or butter-flavored coconut oil if dairy-free)
- ½ cup diced onions
- ½ cup diced celery
- 8 ounces mushrooms, sliced
- 6 cups chicken bone broth, home made or store-bought
- 1 (8-ounce) package cream cheese (Kite Hill brand cream cheese style spread if dairy-free), softened
- 2 cups cooked cubed chicken
- 1 teaspoon fresh thyme, finely chopped
- ½ teaspoon fine sea salt
- ½ teaspoon curry powder
- ½ teaspoon dry mustard
- ½ teaspoon dried parsley
- ½ teaspoon ground black pepper
- chicken cracklings (for crunchy "rice")
- (Makes about 2 cups)
- ½ pound chicken skin and fat
- ½ teaspoon ghee (or lard if dairy-free)
- 2 tablespoons finely diced onions
- 1 small clove garlic, smashed to a paste or minced
- ½ tablespoon fresh sage leaves or other herb of choice, such as thyme
- ½ teaspoon fine sea salt
- ½ teaspoon ground black pepper
- 1 pound bacon, diced, for crunchy "rice"

1. In a stockpot, melt the butter over medium heat.
2. Stir in the onions and celery and sauté for 5 minutes or until soft.
3. Add the mushrooms and sauté for 2 more minutes.
4. Pour in the chicken broth and stir.
5. Bring to a boil, then reduce the heat to low.
6. Add the softened cream cheese and whisk until it is fully incorporated and heated through. Add the chicken and seasonings and simmer, covered, for 1 hour.
7. While the soup is simmering, make the crunchy "rice," starting with the cracklings: Chop the chicken skin into ¼-inch pieces and pat them completely dry with paper towels.
8. Heat the ghee in a medium-sized cast-iron skillet over medium heat.
9. Add the chicken skin pieces, cover, and reduce the heat to low.
10. Cook for 12 to 15 minutes, until there is a layer of liquid fat in the pan.
11. Meanwhile, fry the bacon in a large cast-iron skillet until crispy, about 8 minutes.
12. Remove the bacon from the skillet and set aside until you're ready to serve the soup; reserve the bacon fat for another use.
13. After the chicken fat has cooked on low for 12 to 15 minutes, bring the heat back up to medium and uncover the skillet.
14. Cook the chicken skin pieces for an additional 15 minutes, stirring often, until they start to curl up and there is a lot of fat in the pan.
15. Carefully pour the chicken skin pieces and liquid fat through a colander into a jar.
16. Save the chicken fat for later use—it's a great ketogenic fat—and put the drained chicken skin pieces back in the skillet.
17. To the skillet, add the onions, garlic, and sage and cook over medium heat for another 15 minutes, stirring, until the cracklings are golden brown and crispy.
18. Remove the skillet from the heat.
19. Season the cracklings with the salt and pepper.
20. Ladle the soup into bowls and stir most of the crunchy "rice"—the prepared cracklings and crispy bacon—into the soup.
21. Sprinkle the remaining "rice" on top as a garnish.

Slow Cooker Chipotle Lime Steak Soup

Prep time: 10 minutes|Cook time:4 to 8 hours|Serves 8

- 8 cups beef bone broth, homemade or store-bought
- 1 cup diced onions
- 1 green bell pepper, thinly sliced
- 1 (16-ounce) jar salsa
- ¼ cup diced pickled jalapeños
- 1 chipotle chile pepper in adobo sauce, chopped
- 2½ teaspoons fine sea salt
- 2 teaspoons chili powder
- 1 teaspoon ground cumin
- 1 teaspoon paprika
- ½ teaspoon ground black pepper
- 1 pound boneless beef roast, cut into 2-inch cubes
- 2 limes, halved
- for garnish (optional)
- Fresh cilantro
- Shredded sharp cheddar cheese
- Sour cream
- Lime wedges

1. Combine the broth, onions, bell pepper, salsa, jalapeños, chipotle pepper, salt, and spices in a slow cooker.
2. Place the cubed beef on top of the other ingredients.
3. Cover and cook on low for 8 hours or on high for 4 hours. When the beef is tender, shred the meat with 2 forks. Stir well.
4. Squeeze the lime juice into the slow cooker. Taste and add more salt, if desired.
5. Serve topped with fresh cilantro, cheddar cheese, sour cream, and a lime wedge, if desired.
6. Store extras in an airtight container in the refrigerator for up to 3 days.
7. Reheat in a saucepan over medium heat for a few minutes or until warmed through.

Italian Sausage Soup

Prep time: 10 minutes|Cook time:30 minutes|Serves 6

- 1 tablespoon ghee (or avocado oil if dairy-free)
- 1 pound hot Italian sausages, casings removed
- 6 cups chicken bone broth, homemade or store-bought, divided
- 3 celery stalks, diced
- ½ cup diced onions
- 2 large cloves garlic, minced
- 2 cups cauliflower florets, cut into ½-inch pieces
- 1 cup diced zucchini
- 1 red bell pepper, diced
- 1 teaspoon minced fresh rosemary
- 1 teaspoon minced fresh sage
- 1 teaspoon minced fresh thyme
- ½ teaspoon fine sea salt
- ½ teaspoon ground black pepper
- ½ cup pizza sauce, homemade, or store-bought pizza or marinara sauce
- 1 bay leaf
- Chopped fresh parsley, for garnish (optional)

1. Heat the ghee in a Dutch oven or stockpot over medium heat.
2. Add the sausage and cook for about 6 minutes, breaking it up into small chunks as it browns.
3. When the sausage is fully cooked, remove it from the pot with a slotted spoon. Put it in a bowl and set aside.
4. Add ¼ cup of the chicken broth to the pot and scrape the bottom to deglaze.
5. Add the celery, onions, and garlic and cook, stirring frequently, until the onions are translucent, about 5 minutes.
6. Add the cauliflower, zucchini, bell pepper, herbs, salt, and pepper. Cook, stirring, for another 3 minutes.
7. Add the remaining broth, pizza sauce, and bay leaf.
8. Simmer over medium heat for 8 minutes. Add the cooked sausage and simmer for another 10 minutes. Taste and adjust the seasoning, if desired.
9. Remove and discard the bay leaf.
10. Serve the soup garnished with chopped parsley, if desired.
11. Store extras in an airtight container in the refrigerator for up to 3 days.
12. Reheat in a saucepan over medium heat for a few minutes or until warmed through.

Curried Lentil & Spinach Stew

Prep time: 5 minutes|Cook time:30 minutes|Serves 2

- 1 tbsp extra-virgin olive oil
- 1 tbsp curry powder
- 1 cup homemade chicken or vege-
- table stock
- 1 cup red lentils, soaked
- 1 onion, chopped
- 2 cups butternut squash, cooked peeled and chopped
- 1 cup spinach
- 2 garlic cloves, minced
- 1 tbsp cilantro, finely chopped

1. In a large pot, add the oil, chopped onion and minced garlic, sautéing for 5 minutes on low heat.
2. Add the curry powder and ginger to the onions and cook for 5 minutes.
3. Add the broth and bring to a boil on a high heat.
4. Stir in the lentils, squash and spinach, reduce heat and simmer for a further 20 minutes.
5. Season with pepper to taste and serve with fresh cilantro.

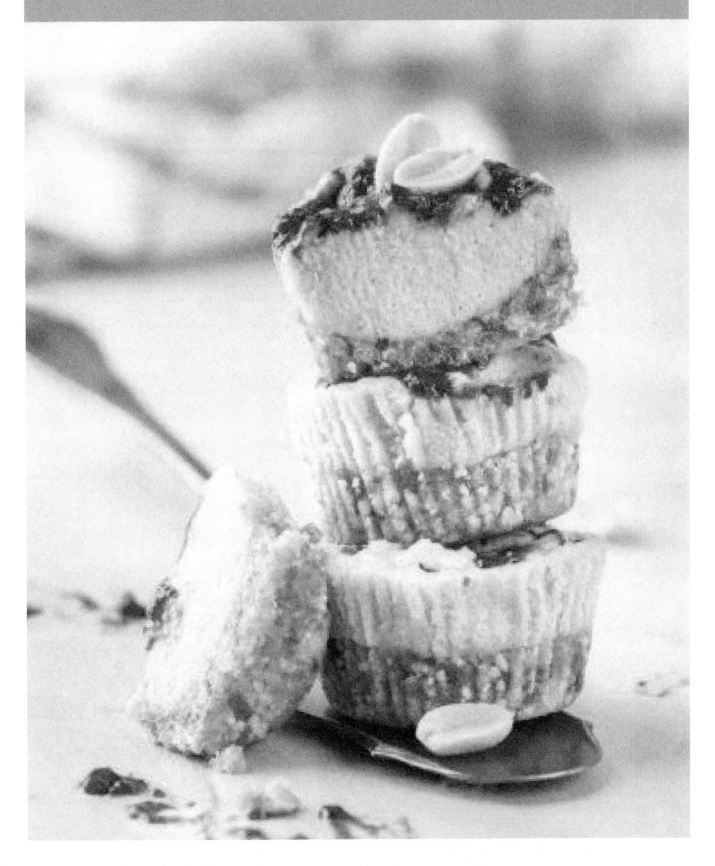

Blackberries And Blueberries

Prep time: 5 minutes|Cook time:20 minutes|Serves 4

- 5 oz [140 g] goat cheese, at room temperature
- 1 1/2 Tbsp honey, plus more for serving
- 1 Tbsp lemon juice
- 1/2 tsp grated orange zest
- Kosher salt
- 2 cups [240 g] blueberries
- 2 cups [240 g] blackberries
- 1/4 cup [30 g] pistachios, chopped

1. Place the goat cheese, honey, lemon juice, orange zest, and a pinch of salt in a medium bowl.
2. Whisk until the goat cheese is fluffy and smooth.
3. Divide the goat cheese mixture among bowls or wineglasses, reserving about four spoonsful.
4. Top each portion with berries, pistachios, and a spoonful of the whipped goat cheese.
5. Drizzle with additional honey. Serve immediately.
6. anything goes
7. Use any kind of fruit for this dessert.
8. And if you are feeling adventurous, fold in your favorite jam or lemon curd for an extra-special treat.

Strawberry-Lime Granita

Prep time: 5 minutes|Cook time:1 hour 45 minutes|Serves 4 to 6

- 1 cup [240 ml] water
- 1/2 cup [100 g] raw cane sugar
- 1 lb [455 g] strawberries, stems removed
- 1/2 cup [120 ml] lime juice

1. Fill a medium bowl with ice water.
2. Combine the 1 cup [240 ml] water and sugar in a small saucepan.
3. Warm over low heat until the sugar is dissolved.
4. Remove the simple syrup from the heat, place the pan in the ice-water bath, and stir to chill rapidly.
5. Alternatively, refrigerate the syrup until chilled, about 3 hours. (Store in an airtight container in the refrigerator for up to 2 weeks.)
6. Reserve four to six strawberries for garnish.
7. Place the remaining strawberries in a blender or food processor.
8. Blend until smooth, then strain through a fine-mesh sieve into a medium bowl to remove the seeds.
9. Add the lime juice and 1/2 cup [120 ml] of the simple syrup to the strawberry juice.
10. Stir and taste, adding more simple syrup if desired.
11. Pour the strawberry mixture into a 13-by-9-by-2-in [33-by-23-by-5-cm] nonstick metal baking pan.
12. Freeze until the mixture is icy around the edges, about 25 minutes.
13. Using a fork, stir the icy portions into the middle of the pan.
14. Continue this process of stirring the icy edges into center every 25 minutes for about 1 1/2 hours, or until the mixture has turned into flaky crystals.
15. Cover tightly and freeze for up to 1 day.
16. To serve, scrape the granita into serving bowls or glasses and garnish with the reserved berries.

Vegan Chocolate Pots De Crème

Prep time: 15 minutes|Cook time:5 minutes|Serves 4 to 6

- 1 lb [455 g] silken tofu, drained
- 2 tsp vanilla extract
- Kosher salt
- 11/2 cups [250 g] semisweet vegan chocolate chips
- 1 tsp maple syrup (optional)
- Chopped strawberries or blueberries for garnish

1. In a medium saucepan, bring 2 in [5 cm] water to a simmer.
2. Place the tofu, vanilla, and 1/4 tsp salt in a blender and puree on low speed until smooth, scraping down the sides with a spatula if needed.
3. When the water is simmering, place the chocolate chips in a medium heatproof bowl that will fit in the saucepan over the simmering water without touching it.
4. Turn the heat to low and melt the chocolate, stirring, until smooth, 2 to 3 minutes.
5. Allow the chocolate to cool slightly, then pour into the blender.
6. Puree until smooth, scraping down the sides if necessary, until the tofu and chocolate are combined.
7. Taste and add the maple syrup if desired. Taste once more and add a pinch of salt if needed.
8. Divide the mixture evenly among six 1/2-cup [120-ml] ramekins.
9. Garnish with berries before serving.

French Meringues

Prep time: 20 minutes|Cook time:2 hours|Serves 30

- 4 large egg whites
- ¼ teaspoon cream of tartar
- ¼ teaspoon sea salt
- ½ cup granulated erythritol-monk fruit blend
- ¼ cup powdered erythritol-monk fruit blend
- ½ teaspoon vanilla extract

1. Preheat the oven to 200°F. Line the baking sheet with parchment paper and set aside.
2. In the large bowl, using an electric mixer on medium, beat the egg whites, cream of tartar, and salt for 1 to 2 minutes, until foamy and the egg whites just begin to turn opaque.
3. Continue to whip the egg whites, adding in the granulated and powdered erythritol–monk fruit blend about 1 teaspoon at a time and scraping the bowl once or twice.
4. Once all the erythritol–monk fruit blend has been added, increase the mixer speed to high and whip for 5 to 7 minutes, until the meringue is glossy and very stiff.
5. Using a rubber spatula, gently fold in the vanilla.
6. Scoop the meringue into the pastry bag fitted with a French star tip and pipe 2-inch-diameter kisses onto the prepared baking sheet.
7. Alternatively, spoon the meringue onto the sheet for a more organic shape.
8. Bake for 2 hours, or until crisp and lightly browned.
9. Allow to cool completely on the cooling rack before serving.
10. Leftovers can be stored in an airtight, nonporous container at room temperature for about 1 week.

Chocolate-Cinnamon Gelato

Prep time: 5 minutes|Cook time:10 minutes|Serves 4 to 6

- 2 tsp cornstarch
- 3 cups [720 ml] Almond Milk or whole milk
- 1/4 tsp kosher salt
- 4 oz [115 g] dark chocolate (70 percent cacao), coarsely chopped
- 1 tsp ground cinnamon
- 1/2 tsp vanilla extract
- Chocolate shavings, crushed walnuts, or crushed fresh raspberries for garnish

1. Put the cornstarch in a small bowl, add 1 Tbsp of the almond milk, and stir with a fork to dissolve the cornstarch.
2. Bring to a simmer over medium heat, then turn the heat to low.
3. Whisk in the cornstarch mixture, sugar, and salt to dissolve. Add the chocolate and cinnamon and whisk until the mixture is completely smooth.
4. Cook, whisking occasionally, until the mixture starts to thicken, about 5 minutes.
5. Pour the milk mixture through a fine-mesh strainer into a large bowl.
6. Stir in the vanilla. Refrigerate until chilled, about 3 hours.
7. Whisk the chilled mixture.
8. Freeze in an ice-cream maker according to the manufacturer's instructions.
9. When ready, the gelato should be the consistency of soft-serve ice cream.
10. Transfer to an airtight container and freeze for up to 1 week.
11. To serve, scoop into serving bowls and garnish as desired.

Cheesecake Fat Bombs

Prep time: 10 minutes|Cook time:1 hour|Serves 30

- 8 ounces full-fat cream cheese, at room temperature
- 8 tablespoons (1 stick) unsalted butter, at room temperature
- 3 tablespoons confectioners' erythritol–monk fruit blend
- 3 tablespoons coconut oil
- ½ teaspoon vanilla extract

1. In the large mixing bowl, using an electric mixer on high, beat the cream cheese and butter for 2 to 3 minutes, until light and fluffy, stopping and scraping the bowl once or twice, as needed.
2. Add the confectioners' erythritol–monk fruit blend, coconut oil, and vanilla and mix until well combined.
3. Scoop the mixture into a pastry bag and pipe into the molds or cupcake liners.
4. Put the molds in the freezer for 1 hour to firm.
5. Pop out the fat bombs to serve.
6. Store in an airtight container in the freezer for up to 3 weeks.

Mini Mocha Bundt Cakes

Prep time: 10 minutes|Cook time:15 minutes|Serves 12

- cakes
- 3 cups blanched almond flour, or 1 cup coconut flour
- ¾ cup unsweetened cocoa powder
- 1 teaspoon baking soda
- ½ teaspoon fine sea salt
- 6 large eggs (12 eggs if using coconut flour)
- 1 cup Swerve confectioners'-style sweetener or equivalent amount of liquid or powdered sweetener
- 3 tablespoons ghee or unsalted butter (or coconut oil if dairy-free), melted but not hot
- 3 tablespoons brewed decaf espresso or other strong brewed decaf coffee (½ cup if using coconut flour)
- 1 teaspoon vanilla extract
- 1½ cups grated zucchini
- glaze
- 1½ cups Swerve confectioners'-style sweetener or equivalent amount of powdered stevia or erythritol
- ¼ cup melted ghee or unsalted butter (or coconut oil if dairy-free)
- 2 tablespoons hot water (for vanilla-flavored glaze) or hot brewed decaf espresso or other strong brewed decaf coffee (for mocha-flavored glaze)
- ½ teaspoon vanilla extract
- ½ cup chopped walnuts or pecans, for garnish (optional)
- special equipment
- 2 (6-well) mini Bundt cake pans

1. Preheat the oven to 350°F. Spray 2 mini Bundt pans with coconut oil spray.
2. To make the cakes, place the flour, cocoa powder, baking soda, and salt in a medium-sized bowl and whisk until blended. In a large bowl, beat the eggs and sweetener with a hand mixer for 2 to 3 minutes, until light and fluffy.
3. Squeeze the water out of the zucchini if it seems wet, then add it to the egg mixture and stir to combine.
4. Add the wet ingredients to the dry ingredients and stir just to combine.
5. Pour the cake batter into the prepared pans, filling each well two-thirds full, and bake for about 15 minutes, until a toothpick inserted into the center of a cake comes out clean.
6. Allow the cakes to cool completely in the pans before removing them.
7. To make the glaze, combine the sweetener with the melted ghee.
8. Stir in the hot water or espresso and vanilla; it should be fairly thick, but thin enough to be stirred with ease.
9. Add more water or espresso if the glaze is too thick; if it's too thin, add more sweetener.
10. Gently spoon the glaze over the cakes, covering the tops. If desired, garnish the cakes with chopped nuts.
11. Store extras in an airtight container in the refrigerator for up to 4 days or in the freezer for up to 1 month.

Sugar Cookies

Prep time: 10 minutes|Cook time:20 minutes|Serves 24

- for the cookies
- 1 cup granulated erythritol–monk fruit blend
- 8 tablespoons (1 stick) unsalted butter, at room temperature
- 1 teaspoon vanilla extract
- 2 large eggs, at room temperature
- ½ cup full-fat sour cream
- 2½ cups finely milled almond flour, sifted
- 1½ teaspoons baking powder
- ¼ teaspoon sea salt
- for the sour cream icing
- 1¼ cups confectioners' erythritol–monk fruit blend
- ½ cup full-fat sour cream
- ½ teaspoon vanilla extract

TO MAKE THE COOKIES

1. Preheat the oven to 350°F.
2. Line the baking sheet with parchment paper and set aside.
3. In the medium bowl, using an electric mixer on high, combine the granulated erythritol–monk fruit blend, butter, and vanilla for 1 to 2 minutes, until light and fluffy, stopping and scraping the bowl once or twice, as needed.
4. Add the eggs, one at a time, to the medium bowl, then add the sour cream.
5. Mix until well incorporated. Next add the almond flour, baking powder, and salt and mix until just combined.
6. Put the dough in the refrigerator and chill for 30 minutes.
7. Drop the dough in tablespoons on the prepared baking sheet evenly spaced about 1 inch apart.
8. Bake the cookies for 15 to 20 minutes, until lightly browned around the edges.
9. Transfer the cookies to a cooling rack to fully cool, 15 to 20 minutes.

TO MAKE THE SOUR CREAM ICING

1. In the small bowl, combine the confectioners' erythritol–monk fruit blend, sour cream, and vanilla.
2. Once the cookies are fully cooled, using a spoon or pastry bag, drizzle the icing on top to serve.
3. Store leftovers in the refrigerator for up to 5 days or freeze for up to 3 weeks.

Iced Gingerbread Cookies

Prep time: 15 minutes|Cook time:30 minutes|Serves 24

- 2 cups brown or golden erythritol–monk fruit blend; less sweet: 1¼ cups
- 3 large eggs
- 4 tablespoons (½ stick) unsalted butter, at room temperature
- 1 tablespoon molasses or 1 teaspoon molasses extract (optional)
- 1 teaspoon vanilla extract
- 4 tablespoons ground cinnamon
- 3 tablespoons ground ginger
- ½ teaspoon ground nutmeg
- ¼ teaspoon ground cloves
- 3 cups finely milled almond flour
- 1 tablespoon psyllium husk powder
- 1½ teaspoons baking powder
- ¼ teaspoon salt
- ¼ cup confectioners' erythritol–monk fruit blend
- 1 tablespoon heavy (whipping) cream

1. Preheat the oven to 325°F.
2. Line the baking sheet with parchment paper and set aside.
3. In the large bowl, using an electric mixer on high, beat the brown erythritol–monk fruit blend, eggs, butter, molasses (if using), and vanilla until fully incorporated, stopping and scraping the bowl once or twice, as needed.
4. Add the cinnamon, ginger, nutmeg, and cloves to the mixture and stir to combine.
5. Add the almond flour, psyllium powder, baking powder, and salt and beat on medium high until well incorporated.
6. Place the dough between two sheets of parchment paper and flatten with a rolling pin.
7. Chill the dough in the refrigerator for 30 minutes.
8. Using a small cookie cutter or small-mouthed glass jar, cut the dough into cookies and place them about 1 inch apart, evenly spaced, on the prepared baking sheet.
9. Bake for 12 to 15 minutes, until golden brown.
10. Allow them to cool completely on the cooling rack, 15 to 20 minutes.
11. In the small bowl, combine the confectioners' erythritol–monk fruit blend with the heavy cream 1 teaspoon at a time to make the icing.
12. The icing should have a runny consistency.
13. Decorate the cooled cookies using either a pastry bag for fine detail or drizzle the icing on using a fork for a quick, fuss-free decorated cookie.
14. Store leftovers in an airtight container in the refrigerator for up to 5 days or freeze for up to 3 weeks.

Malted Milk Ball Cheesecake

Prep time: 10 minutes|Cook time:1 hour|Serves 16

- crust
- 3½ tablespoons unsalted butter (or coconut oil if dairy-free), plus extra for the pan
- 1½ ounces unsweetened chocolate, finely chopped
- ⅓ cup Swerve confectioners'-style sweetener or equivalent amount of liquid or powdered sweetener
- 1 teaspoon stevia glycerite
- 1 large egg, beaten
- 2 teaspoons ground cinnamon
- Seeds scraped from 1 vanilla bean (about 8 inches long), or 1 teaspoon vanilla extract
- ¼ teaspoon fine sea salt
- filling
- 6 (8-ounce) packages cream cheese (Kite Hill brand cream cheese style spread if dairy-free)
- ¾ cup Swerve confectioners'-style sweetener or equivalent amount of liquid or powdered sweetener
- ½ cup maca powder
- Seeds scraped from 1 vanilla bean (about 8 inches long), or 1 teaspoon vanilla extract
- 3 large eggs
- ganache
- 1 cup heavy cream (or full-fat coconut milk if dairy-free)
- ⅓ cup Swerve confectioners'-style sweetener or equivalent amount of liquid or powdered sweetener
- 2 ounces unsweetened chocolate, finely chopped
- Seeds scraped from 1 vanilla bean (about 8 inches long), or 1 teaspoon vanilla extract
- ⅛ teaspoon fine sea salt
- special equipment
- inch springform pan

1. Preheat the oven to 350°F.
2. Grease an 8-inch springform pan, then line it with parchment paper and grease the paper.
3. Mix together the crust ingredients, then press the crust mixture into the prepared pan.
4. Combine the cream cheese, sweetener, maca powder, and vanilla with a hand mixer until blended.
5. Add the eggs one at a time, mixing on low after each addition, just until blended.
6. Pour the batter on top of the crust in the springform pan.
7. Set up a water bath: Wrap aluminum foil entirely around the bottom and halfway up the sides of the springform pan to prevent water from leaking into the removable bottom of the pan.
8. Place the wrapped pan inside a roasting pan (or any baking dish with sides) and place the pans in the oven. Pour hot water into the roasting pan so that it comes halfway up the sides of the springform pan. (Note: A water bath helps cook the cheesecake evenly; however, the cheesecake can be baked without it.
9. See the note on here if you choose not to use a water bath.) Bake for 1 hour or until the center of the cheesecake is almost set.
10. Let the cake cool completely in the pan before removing the outer ring. Refrigerate the cheesecake overnight.
11. Just before serving, make the ganache: Bring the cream and sweetener to a simmer in a saucepan over medium heat.
12. Remove from the heat and add the chopped chocolate, vanilla, and salt. Stir, then allow to sit for 3 minutes.
13. Stir again until completely smooth.
14. Pour the ganache over the chilled cheesecake, then place the cake in the refrigerator to set for 10 minutes before serving.
15. Store extras in an airtight container in the refrigerator for up to 4 days.

Honey Panna Cotta

Prep time: 10 minutes|Cook time:4 to 8 hours|Serves 6

- 21/2 cups [600 ml] canned unsweetened coconut milk
- 2 tsp gelatin
- 1/4 cup [60 ml] honey
- 1 vanilla bean, split and seeds scraped
- Kosher salt
- blackberry-lime sauce
- 2 cups [240 g] blackberries
- Finely grated zest of 1/2 lime, plus 2 tsp lime juice
- 1 tsp raw cane sugar

1. Place 1/2 cup [120 ml] of the coconut milk in a small bowl.
2. Sprinkle the gelatin over the top and allow it to sit for about 2 minutes.
3. Place the remaining 2 cups [480 ml] coconut milk, the honey, vanilla bean and its seeds, and a pinch of salt in a medium saucepan.
4. Warm over low heat, whisking occasionally, until bubbles form around the edge of the pan.
5. Remove from the heat and let the mixture steep for 5 minutes.
6. Pour the coconut milk mixture through a fine-mesh strainer into a large bowl. Discard the vanilla bean.
7. Whisk the gelatin mixture slowly into the warm coconut mixture until there are no lumps of gelatin.
8. Divide evenly among six 1/2-cup [120-ml] ramekins or wineglasses.
9. Cover and refrigerate until set, at least 4 hours or up to overnight.
10. To make the blackberry-lime sauce: Place the blackberries, lime zest, lime juice, and sugar in a medium bowl.
11. Using a fork or pastry blender, gently mash the berries, leaving some large pieces of berry while allowing some of the juices to make a sauce.
12. Set aside for at least 10 minutes, or cover and refrigerate up to overnight.
13. Spoon the sauce over each chilled panna cotta. Serve immediately.

Cannoli Mini Cheese Balls

Prep time: 10 minutes|Cook time:30 minutes|Serves 8

- cannoli balls
- 1 (8-ounce) package cream cheese or mascarpone cheese (Kite Hill brand cream cheese style spread if dairy-free), softened
- ½ cup ricotta cheese (or Kite Hill brand cream cheese style spread, softened, if dairy-free)
- ½ cup Swerve confectioners'-style sweetener or equivalent amount of liquid or powdered sweetener
- 1 teaspoon ground cinnamon
- chocolate chunks
- 1 cup (2 sticks) unsalted butter (or coconut oil if dairy-free), melted
- ¾ cup Swerve confectioners'-style sweetener or equivalent amount of liquid or powdered sweetener
- 1 teaspoon almond extract (omit for nut-free)
- 1 teaspoon vanilla extract
- ¼ teaspoon fine sea salt
- chocolate drizzle
- ¼ cup heavy cream (or full-fat coconut milk if dairy-free)
- 1 ounce unsweetened chocolate, finely chopped
- 2 tablespoons Swerve confectioners'-style sweetener or equivalent amount of liquid or powdered sweetener
- Seeds scraped from 1 vanilla bean (about 8 inches long), or 1 teaspoon vanilla extract

1. To make the cannoli balls, place the cream cheese, ricotta, sweetener, and cinnamon in a medium-sized bowl.
2. Mix well with a hand mixer. Using your hands, form the mixture into eight 2-inch balls and place on a rimmed baking sheet or tray.
3. Cover and refrigerate for at least 30 minutes, until firm.
4. To make the chocolate chunks, place a piece of parchment paper in a 9-inch pie pan.
5. Place all the ingredients for the chunks in a blender and pulse until smooth.
6. Taste and adjust the sweetness to your liking.
7. Pour the mixture onto the parchment and place the pie pan in the refrigerator or freezer to set, about 20 minutes in the fridge or 10 minutes in the freezer.
8. Once hard, chop the chocolate into small pieces and place them in a shallow bowl.
9. To make the drizzle, place the cream, chopped chocolate, and sweetener in a double boiler or in a heat-safe bowl set over a pan of simmering water.
10. Heat on low, stirring, just until the chocolate melts. Remove from the heat and stir in the vanilla.
11. Place in the refrigerator to cool for 8 minutes or until thickened, but still a bit warm; if the chocolate hardens too much, return it to the double boiler and reheat gently.
12. Remove the cream cheese balls from the fridge and roll them in the chocolate pieces.
13. Drizzle the chocolate-coated balls with the chocolate drizzle.
14. Store extras in an airtight container in the refrigerator for up to 4 days.

Mint Chocolate Whoopie Pies

Prep time: 10 minutes|Cook time:12 minutes|Serves 6

- 1¼ cups blanched almond flour, or ½ cup coconut flour
- ¼ cup unsweetened cocoa powder
- ½ teaspoon baking soda
- ¼ teaspoon fine sea salt
- ¼ cup (½ stick) unsalted butter or coconut oil, softened, plus extra for the pans
- ⅓ cup Swerve confectioners'-style sweetener or equivalent amount of liquid or powdered sweetener
- 3 large eggs (6 eggs and ¼ cup unsweetened almond milk if using coconut flour)
- 1 teaspoon mint extract
- filling
- ¾ cup (1½ sticks) unsalted butter, softened
- ¾ cup Swerve confectioners'-style sweetener or equivalent amount of liquid or powdered sweetener
- 1 tablespoon heavy cream
- 1 teaspoon mint extract
- chocolate drizzle
- ¼ cup heavy cream
- 2 tablespoons Swerve confectioners'-style sweetener or equivalent amount of liquid or powdered sweetener
- ½ ounce unsweetened chocolate, finely chopped
- ½ teaspoon vanilla extract
- Fresh mint leaves, for garnish (optional)
- special equipment
- well whoopie pie pan or muffin top pan

1. Preheat the oven to 325°F. Grease a 12-well whoopie pie pan (or muffin top pan).
2. In a mixing bowl, whisk together the flour, cocoa powder, baking soda, and salt until blended.
3. In a separate bowl, beat the butter, sweetener, eggs, and extract with a hand mixer until smooth. Stir the wet ingredients into the flour mixture.
4. Spoon the batter into the prepared pan, filling each well about two-thirds full.
5. Bake for 12 minutes or until a toothpick inserted into the center of a pie comes out clean. Allow to cool in the pan.
6. Meanwhile, make the filling: Using the hand mixer, cream the butter, cream cheese, and sweetener in a medium-sized bowl.
7. Add the heavy cream to thin it out a little, then add the mint extract and mix to combine. Set the filling aside.
8. Heat on low, stirring, just until the chocolate is melted. Remove from the heat and stir in the vanilla. Taste and add more sweetener, if desired.
9. To assemble the whoopie pies, place one pie flat side up on a plate.
10. Place 2 tablespoons of filling on the pie, then top with another pie. Repeat with the rest of the pies and filling.
11. Drizzle the chocolate over each whoopie pie.
12. Serve garnished with mint leaves, if desired.
13. Store extras in an airtight container in the refrigerator for up to 4 days.

Appendix 1 Measurement Conversion Chart

Volume Equivalents (Dry)

US STANDARD	METRIC (APPROXIMATE)
1/8 teaspoon	0.5 mL
1/4 teaspoon	1 mL
1/2 teaspoon	2 mL
3/4 teaspoon	4 mL
1 teaspoon	5 mL
1 tablespoon	15 mL
1/4 cup	59 mL
1/2 cup	118 mL
3/4 cup	177 mL
1 cup	235 mL
2 cups	475 mL
3 cups	700 mL
4 cups	1 L

Volume Equivalents (Liquid)

US STANDARD	US STANDARD (OUNCES)	METRIC (APPROXIMATE)
2 tablespoons	1 fl.oz.	30 mL
1/4 cup	2 fl.oz.	60 mL
1/2 cup	4 fl.oz.	120 mL
1 cup	8 fl.oz.	240 mL
1 1/2 cup	12 fl.oz.	355 mL
2 cups or 1 pint	16 fl.oz.	475 mL
4 cups or 1 quart	32 fl.oz.	1 L
1 gallon	128 fl.oz.	4 L

Temperatures Equivalents

FAHRENHEIT(F)	CELSIUS(C) APPROXIMATE
225 °F	107 °C
250 °F	120 ° °C
275 °F	135 °C
300 °F	150 °C
325 °F	160 °C
350 °F	180 °C
375 °F	190 °C
400 °F	205 °C
425 °F	220 °C
450 °F	235 °C
475 °F	245 °C
500 °F	260 °C

Weight Equivalents

US STANDARD	METRIC (APPROXIMATE)
1 ounce	28 g
2 ounces	57 g
5 ounces	142 g
10 ounces	284 g
15 ounces	425 g
16 ounces (1 pound)	455 g
1.5 pounds	680 g
2 pounds	907 g

Appendix 2 The Dirty Dozen and Clean Fifteen

The Environmental Working Group (EWG) is a nonprofit, nonpartisan organization dedicated to protecting human health and the environment Its mission is to empower people to live healthier lives in a healthier environment. This organization publishes an annual list of the twelve kinds of produce, in sequence, that have the highest amount of pesticide residue-the Dirty Dozen-as well as a list of the fifteen kinds ofproduce that have the least amount of pesticide residue-the Clean Fifteen.

THE DIRTY DOZEN	
The 2016 Dirty Dozen includes the following produce. These are considered among the year's most important produce to buy organic:	
Strawberries	Spinach
Apples	Tomatoes
Nectarines	Bell peppers
Peaches	Cherry tomatoes
Celery	Cucumbers
Grapes	Kale/collard greens
Cherries	Hot peppers

The Dirty Dozen list contains two additional itemskale/ collard greens and hot peppers-because they tend to contain trace levels of highly hazardous pesticides.

THE CLEAN FIFTEEN	
The least critical to buy organically are the Clean Fifteen list. The following are on the 2016 list:	
Avocados	Papayas
Corn	Kiw
Pineapples	Eggplant
Cabbage	Honeydew
Sweet peas	Grapefruit
Onions	Cantaloupe
Asparagus	Cauliflower
Mangos	

Some of the sweet corn sold in the United States are made from genetically engineered (GE) seedstock. Buy organic varieties of these crops to avoid GE produce.

Appendix 3 Index

PATRICIA J. SCHWARTZ

Printed in Great Britain
by Amazon

24352302R00051